The Ayurvedic Path to Wellness

Dedication

This book is dedicated to the ancient wisdom of Ayurveda and to all those who seek a path towards holistic well-being. It is a tribute to the countless individuals throughout history who have practiced and preserved this timeless system of healing. It's also dedicated to the modern seekers—those bravely navigating the complexities of modern life while yearning for a more balanced and fulfilling existence. May this work serve as a guiding light, illuminating the path to self-discovery and empowerment, fostering a journey toward a healthier, happier, and more harmonious life. This is for those who believe in the power of nature, the wisdom of the body, and the transformative potential of self-care. To the courageous individuals who embrace the principles of Ayurveda and integrate them into their lives, transforming their health and well-being, this book is offered with gratitude and respect. This dedication extends to all those who have shared their stories, experiences, and insights, enriching our understanding of this ancient practice and inspiring others to embark on their own transformative journeys. It is a testament to the enduring power of holistic health and the enduring human spirit. It is a testament to the power of resilience, self-compassion, and the unwavering pursuit of a balanced and joyful existence.

Preface

In a world characterized by relentless pace and technological advancements, the ancient wisdom of Ayurveda offers a refreshing perspective on health and well-being. This book aims to bridge the gap between this timeless system of healing and the modern world, providing a practical and accessible guide to integrating Ayurvedic principles into daily life. It is not merely a collection of recipes and routines; it's a journey of self-discovery, inviting readers to explore their unique constitution, understand their imbalances, and cultivate a deeper connection with their bodies and minds. We have endeavored to present complex Ayurvedic concepts in a clear and engaging manner, using relatable examples, stunning visuals, and a conversational tone. We believe that the key to achieving optimal health lies in understanding the interconnectedness of mind, body, and spirit, and Ayurveda provides the framework for nurturing this interconnectedness. This book is designed to empower you to take an active role in your health journey, equipping you with the knowledge and tools to create a personalized wellness plan that resonates with your individual needs and preferences. We encourage you to approach this book as a companion on your transformative journey, a resource that you can revisit and refer to as you embark on your exploration of the ancient path to holistic wellness. Remember, the journey to optimal health is a personal one, and this book serves as a guide, supporting and empowering you every step of the way. Embrace the process, celebrate your successes, and be kind to yourself along the way. Your health and well-being are worth the investment.

Introduction

Welcome to the world of Ayurveda, an ancient Indian system of medicine that offers a holistic approach to health and well-being. For thousands of years, Ayurveda has guided individuals towards a life of balance and harmony, emphasizing the interconnectedness of mind, body, and spirit. This comprehensive guide will unveil the secrets of this timeless system, empowering you to take control of your health and create a life of vitality and joy. We will explore the fundamental principles of Ayurveda, introducing the three doshas—Vata, Pitta, and Kapha—and their influence on your physical and mental health. Through detailed explanations and a user-friendly Dosha Wheel, you will learn to identify your predominant dosha and understand its unique characteristics. The core of this book focuses on personalized wellness plans tailored to each dosha, emphasizing the importance of dietary balance, mindful movement, and stress management. Detailed Ayurvedic meal plans, mouth-watering recipes, and visually appealing exercise charts are provided, categorized by dosha to help you nourish your body and harmonize your mind. We'll delve into the six tastes and their impact on your doshas, along with seasonal dietary adjustments to ensure optimal balance throughout the year. This book also explores the significance of daily routines (Dinacharya) and the role of Panchakarma (Ayurvedic detox) and Rasayana (rejuvenation therapies) in maintaining equilibrium. We'll examine the integration of Ayurveda with modern medicine, backing its claims with scientific evidence and real-life success stories. Our 30-day Ayurvedic wellness plan will provide weekly guidance, recipes, exercises, and self-care practices to empower you on your journey to a healthier, more balanced life. With vibrant visuals, including recipe photos and an herb guide, this book will provide a holistic and practical approach to enhancing your overall well-being. Embrace this opportunity to embark on a transformative journey towards a healthier and more balanced life – a life lived in harmony with yourself and the world around you.

Understanding the Philosophy of Ayurveda

Ayurveda, meaning "the science of life," is a holistic healing system originating in ancient India. Unlike Western medicine, which often focuses on treating symptoms, Ayurveda takes a preventative and personalized approach, aiming to maintain overall well-being and prevent disease before it arises. This ancient wisdom views health not simply as the absence of illness, but as a state of dynamic equilibrium – a harmonious balance between mind, body, and spirit. This equilibrium, crucial for optimal health, is achieved through a profound understanding and nurturing of the individual's unique constitution. At its heart lies the principle of
prakriti
, which refers to one's inherent nature or constitution, determined by the balance of three fundamental energies known as
doshas
.

The core philosophy of Ayurveda revolves around the concept of balance, or
equilibrium
. This balance isn't static; it's a dynamic interplay of forces constantly striving for harmony. When this equilibrium is disrupted, it creates an imbalance, leading to the manifestation of disease.
Ayurveda's goal is to restore this balance, not just to treat the disease itself. The system's approach involves understanding the root cause of the imbalance, rather than merely addressing the surface symptoms. This holistic approach considers the individual's physical, mental, and emotional states, recognizing the interconnectedness of these aspects in the overall state of health.

Understanding the intricate interplay of these elements is crucial in achieving and maintaining optimal health within the Ayurvedic framework. Disease isn't viewed as a separate entity, but rather as a manifestation of an imbalance within this intricate system. Therefore, treatment involves restoring the natural harmony of the body and mind, facilitating the body's innate healing capabilities. This individualized approach contrasts sharply with conventional medicine's frequently generalized treatment plans. Ayurveda tailors treatments and preventative measures to an individual's unique constitution, ensuring a more personalized and effective approach to wellness.

A key element of this personalized approach is the concept of *Prakriti*, which represents the individual's innate constitution or blueprint. This constitution, determined at conception, is a unique blend of the three doshas: Vata, Pitta, and Kapha. Understanding one's Prakriti is fundamental to achieving optimal health in Ayurveda. It serves as a roadmap to understand individual strengths, weaknesses, predispositions to disease, and the best approaches to maintain balance. By recognizing your Prakriti, you gain invaluable insight into your body's natural tendencies, enabling you to make conscious choices that support your unique constitution.

The three doshas – Vata, Pitta, and Kapha – represent the fundamental energies that govern physiological and psychological functions. These doshas aren't merely physical qualities but rather energetic principles that influence every aspect of our being, from our digestion and metabolism to our emotions and thoughts. Vata, characterized by air and ether, governs movement, creativity, and communication. Individuals with a predominantly Vata constitution tend to be energetic, creative, and adaptable, but can also be prone to anxiety, insomnia, and digestive issues if their Vata is imbalanced.

Pitta, associated with fire and water, governs metabolism, transformation, and digestion. Those with a predominantly

Pitta constitution are often intelligent, ambitious, and assertive, but can be prone to irritability, inflammation, and digestive upset if their Pitta becomes imbalanced. They are driven individuals but may need to prioritize managing stress and avoiding overheating. Finally, Kapha, associated with earth and water, governs structure, stability, and lubrication. Individuals with a predominantly Kapha constitution are usually calm, compassionate, and stable but can be prone to weight gain, sluggishness, and respiratory issues if their Kapha becomes imbalanced. They benefit from activities that promote movement and lightness.

The Ayurvedic approach emphasizes preventative measures, focusing on maintaining equilibrium before disease manifests. This approach often involves dietary adjustments, lifestyle modifications, and herbal remedies tailored to an individual's unique doshic constitution. The goal is to enhance the body's inherent healing capacity and maintain a harmonious state of balance. Ayurveda goes beyond simply treating the symptoms; it aims to address the root cause of the imbalance.

Understanding the interplay of the doshas and their influence on our physical and mental well-being is crucial. An imbalance in any of the doshas can manifest in various symptoms, ranging from digestive problems and sleep disturbances to emotional imbalances and chronic diseases. Ayurveda provides various tools and techniques to identify these imbalances and restore harmony. These include dietary adjustments, lifestyle modifications, herbal remedies, and specific therapies such as Panchakarma (a comprehensive detoxification process) and Rasayana (rejuvenation therapies).

The concept of the Panchamahabhutas, the five great elements – ether (akasha), air (vayu), fire (agni), water (jala), and earth (prithvi) – forms the foundation of Ayurveda's understanding of the human body and its interaction with the environment. These five elements are not just physical substances but fundamental energies that constitute everything in the universe, including our bodies. Each dosha is a unique combination of these five elements, creating a dynamic interplay of energies within the individual.

Vata, for instance, is predominantly composed of air and ether, giving it its dynamic and mobile nature. Pitta, with its fire and water components, explains its transformative and metabolic properties. Kapha, with earth and water, embodies its grounding and stabilizing qualities. Understanding the elemental composition of the doshas helps in identifying imbalances and applying appropriate treatments to restore harmony. By recognizing how these elements manifest in our bodies and interact with our environment, we can make conscious choices to support our unique constitution and enhance our overall well-being.

The philosophy of Ayurveda extends beyond the physical body. It recognizes the importance of mental and emotional well-being, emphasizing the interconnectedness of mind, body, and spirit. Stress, for example, is seen not merely as a modern affliction but as a significant factor that disrupts the delicate balance of the doshas, contributing to various health problems. Ayurveda offers various stress-management techniques, including meditation, yoga, and herbal remedies, to help restore balance and promote mental clarity. The emphasis on mindfulness and self-awareness plays a pivotal role in achieving this balance.

Ayurveda promotes a lifestyle that integrates various aspects of well-being, including mindful eating, regular exercise, adequate sleep, and stress management. These practices, collectively known as
dinacharya
(daily routine), are

designed to support the natural rhythms of the body and maintain doshic balance. The daily routine isn't a rigid set of rules but rather a flexible framework adapted to individual needs and preferences. The ultimate goal is to create a lifestyle that promotes balance, vitality, and longevity. This holistic approach encourages a proactive rather than reactive approach to health, emphasizing prevention and self-care.

Adopting an Ayurvedic lifestyle isn't about following strict rules but about making conscious choices that support your unique constitution and promote balance. It is a journey of self-discovery and self-care, guided by the ancient wisdom of Ayurveda. The emphasis is on gradual integration and sustainable changes, fostering a harmonious relationship between the individual and their environment. The beauty of Ayurveda lies in its adaptability and personalization, making it a holistic system accessible to all who seek a path towards optimal health and well-being. It's a journey of understanding your body, honoring its inherent wisdom, and living in harmony with the natural world.

Vata Pitta and Kapha

Understanding the interplay of these three doshas is fundamental to Ayurvedic practice. They are not merely static entities but dynamic energies that constantly fluctuate based on various internal and external factors, such as diet, lifestyle, season, and emotional state. The key to Ayurvedic wellness lies in identifying your unique doshic constitution (Prakriti) and maintaining a balance amongst these energies. An imbalance, or
Vikriti
, can lead to various health issues.

Vata, the first dosha, is associated with the elements of air and ether (space). Think of the wind, the rustling leaves, the movement of the air—this is the essence of Vata. It governs movement, both physical and mental. Individuals with a predominantly Vata constitution are often characterized by their quick wit, creativity, and adaptability. However, an excess of Vata can manifest as anxiety, insomnia, constipation, dry skin, and erratic energy levels. Imagine a gust of wind—unpredictable, swift, and potentially disruptive. That's the nature of Vata when out of balance. Maintaining equilibrium for a Vata-dominant individual requires a focus on routines, grounding practices, warm foods, and a calming environment. Think warm baths, regular sleep schedules, and foods that are rich in fats and oils—to counteract the drying effects of Vata's airy nature. Nourishing foods like warm soups, stews, and cooked vegetables provide a sense of stability and warmth. Regular massage with warm sesame oil can help to ground and soothe the nervous system.

Pitta, the second dosha, is associated with the elements of fire and water. It governs transformation, metabolism, and digestion. Think of the sun's warmth, the digestive fire within your body, the transformative power of heat—this is the energy of Pitta. Those with a predominantly Pitta constitution are often intelligent, assertive, ambitious, and passionate. However, an excess of Pitta can lead to inflammation, anger, heartburn, ulcers, and skin irritations. Picture a fire—powerful, transformative, but also capable of causing destruction if uncontrolled. That's Pitta's essence when out of balance. Balancing Pitta involves cooling measures, such as incorporating cooling foods into the diet, maintaining a calm demeanor, and avoiding excessive exertion. Think of cooling fruits and vegetables like cucumber, watermelon, and mint. Avoiding spicy foods, excessive sunlight, and stressful situations are also crucial. Regular exercise is beneficial, but it should be moderate, avoiding intense workouts that overheat the body.

Kapha, the third dosha, is associated with the elements of earth and water. It governs structure, stability, and lubrication. Think of the earth's grounding presence, the slow and steady growth of plants, the lubricant qualities of water—this is the essence of Kapha. Those with a predominantly Kapha constitution are often loving, compassionate, stable, and grounded. However, an excess of Kapha can manifest as sluggishness, weight gain, mucus congestion, and a tendency towards depression. Envision the earth—stable, fertile, but prone to stagnation if not properly cultivated. That's Kapha when out of balance. Restoring balance for a Kapha-dominant individual requires stimulating activities and foods with warming, light, and pungent qualities. The key is to encourage movement and prevent stagnation in both the body and the mind. Light exercises such as yoga and brisk walking are beneficial. Incorporating spices like ginger, cinnamon, and black pepper into the diet can enhance metabolism and promote digestion. Avoiding heavy, rich foods and limiting dairy consumption can also contribute to maintaining a balanced Kapha dosha.

Each dosha has its unique qualities and tendencies, and most individuals possess a combination of all three. However, one dosha typically predominates, forming the foundation of their constitution. Understanding your predominant dosha helps you make informed choices about diet, lifestyle, and self-care practices to maintain balance and promote optimal health.

It is important to note that these are general characteristics, and individual experiences may vary. There are various nuances within each dosha type. For example, a Vata individual can lean towards a more Vata-Pitta or Vata-Kapha constitution, influencing their specific needs and tendencies. Similarly, Pitta can have subtle variations leaning towards Vata-Pitta or Pitta-Kapha, and Kapha can present as Kapha-Vata or Kapha-Pitta. This highlights the complexity of the Ayurvedic system and the need for a personalized approach. A thorough assessment by a qualified Ayurvedic practitioner can provide a deeper understanding of your unique constitution and guide you towards a tailored wellness plan.

Determining your predominant dosha can be a fascinating journey of self-discovery. While a consultation with an Ayurvedic practitioner is ideal for an accurate assessment, you can gain valuable insights through self-observation and a simple questionnaire. Pay attention to your physical and mental characteristics, your preferences in food and activity, and your typical reactions to seasonal changes and stress. Consider the following questions:

Physical Build:
Are you slender and light-boned (Vata), medium build and muscular (Pitta), or robust and larger (Kapha)?
Energy Levels:
Are you energetic but prone to fatigue (Vata), energetic and intense (Pitta), or steady and enduring

(Kapha)?

Digestion:
Do you have irregular digestion (Vata), strong digestion but prone to heartburn (Pitta), or slow digestion (Kapha)?

Sleep Patterns:
Do you have difficulty sleeping or erratic sleep patterns (Vata), generally good sleep but prone to vivid dreams (Pitta), or long and deep sleep (Kapha)?

Mental Characteristics:
Are you creative, quick-witted, and adaptable (Vata), assertive, ambitious, and focused (Pitta), or calm, compassionate, and grounded (Kapha)?

Skin:
Is your skin dry and prone to wrinkles (Vata), warm and sensitive (Pitta), or oily and prone to acne (Kapha)? **Hair:** Is your hair fine, dry and brittle (Vata), fine to medium texture, oily (Pitta), or thick, oily and wavy (Kapha)?

By honestly answering these questions and reflecting on your overall constitution, you can begin to identify your predominant dosha. Numerous online resources and books offer more detailed questionnaires to further refine this assessment. However, it is important to remember that this self-assessment provides only a preliminary understanding. A proper diagnosis and personalized treatment plan should always be sought from a qualified Ayurvedic practitioner.

The three doshas—Vata, Pitta, and Kapha—are not simply personality types; they represent fundamental bio-energies that govern the physiological and psychological aspects of an individual's being. Understanding their interaction and identifying your predominant dosha is the cornerstone of Ayurvedic wellness. It paves the way for a personalized approach to maintaining equilibrium and preventing illness, fostering a life of vitality, balance, and harmony. By paying close attention to your individual constitution and its subtle shifts, you embark on a transformative journey towards a healthier, happier, and more fulfilled existence. Remember that Ayurveda is a journey of self-discovery, continuous learning, and adaptation. The more you understand your unique constitution and how it responds to various factors, the better equipped you'll be to maintain your optimal state of balance. Embrace this ancient wisdom, and let it guide you towards a holistic and integrated approach to wellness. By consciously living in accordance with the rhythms of nature and the subtle intelligence of your own body, you will unlock the potential for enduring health and well-being. The journey to understand your doshas and utilize this knowledge is a lifelong commitment to self-care, a testament to the wisdom of Ayurveda, and a cornerstone of a truly fulfilling life.

A Harmonious Integration

The enduring relevance of Ayurveda in the 21st century lies not only in its rich history and holistic approach but also in its growing validation by modern scientific research. While Ayurveda's origins predate modern scientific methodologies, a wealth of contemporary studies are beginning to unravel the intricate mechanisms behind its effectiveness. This convergence of ancient wisdom and modern science offers a compelling narrative for those seeking a path to holistic well-being that is both grounded in tradition and supported by evidence.

One of the most significant areas of convergence lies in the understanding of the doshas. While Ayurveda describes Vata, Pitta, and Kapha as fundamental bio-energies, modern science can correlate these doshas with physiological processes and psychological predispositions. For instance, Vata's characteristics – characterized by lightness, dryness, and movement – can be understood through the lens of neurotransmitters and the autonomic nervous system. Individuals with a predominantly Vata constitution often exhibit a faster metabolism, a tendency towards anxiety, and a predisposition to conditions like constipation and insomnia. Modern research into neurotransmitters, such as dopamine and serotonin, offers insights into the mechanisms that underpin these characteristics, providing a scientific framework for understanding Vata imbalances and their treatment.

Similarly, Pitta, associated with fire and transformation, can be linked to metabolic processes and inflammatory responses. Its characteristics – intensity, heat, and sharpness– are reflected in individuals with a higher body temperature, a strong digestive system, and a tendency towards quick decision-making. However, an imbalance in Pitta can manifest as inflammation, digestive issues like heartburn and ulcers, and even skin conditions like acne. Contemporary research in immunology and inflammatory pathways aligns with the Ayurvedic understanding of Pitta imbalances, providing a scientific basis for interventions like dietary modifications and lifestyle adjustments.

Kapha, representing earth and water elements, relates to structure, stability, and lubrication. Individuals with a predominant Kapha constitution typically exhibit a slower metabolism, a calm temperament, and a strong immune system. However, an excess of Kapha can lead to sluggishness, weight gain, and respiratory issues. Modern research on metabolic processes, particularly the role of hormones and body composition, provides valuable insights into Kapha imbalances and their management. Studies on body fat distribution and metabolic rate correlate with the Ayurvedic understanding of Kapha's influence on these physiological processes.

Beyond the doshas, many Ayurvedic practices are finding scientific support. The emphasis on dietary balance, for example, aligns perfectly with modern nutritional science. Ayurveda's emphasis on whole foods, seasonal eating, and the six tastes – sweet, sour, salty, bitter, pungent, and astringent – finds echoes in the current emphasis on balanced diets rich in fruits, vegetables, and whole grains. The science behind the benefits of specific foods – for instance, the anti-inflammatory properties of turmeric or the digestive benefits of ginger – are constantly being investigated and affirmed through modern research, lending scientific credence to traditional Ayurvedic recommendations.

Ayurvedic herbal remedies are another area attracting considerable scientific interest. Many traditional Ayurvedic herbs are now undergoing rigorous scientific scrutiny, revealing their potent pharmacological properties. Turmeric, for example, long celebrated for its anti-inflammatory and antioxidant properties, is now being studied extensively for its potential in preventing and treating various diseases, including cancer and Alzheimer's. Similarly, research into Ashwagandha, a potent adaptogen, reveals its stress-reducing and immune-boosting properties. This scientific validation of traditional Ayurvedic remedies underscores the rich potential of integrating these natural therapies into modern healthcare.

The Ayurvedic concept of Dinacharya, the daily routine, resonates with modern understanding of circadian rhythms and their impact on health and well-being. The emphasis on regularity in sleep, meal timings, and physical activity aligns with modern scientific research highlighting the importance of these factors in maintaining hormonal balance, optimizing metabolic functions, and promoting overall health. Moreover, the integration of yoga and meditation, core components of Ayurvedic practice, has been extensively researched for their stress-reducing and mood-enhancing properties. These practices are now recommended by healthcare professionals worldwide for their impact on physical and mental health, highlighting the synergistic integration of Ayurvedic wisdom and modern scientific understanding.

Ayurveda's emphasis on Panchakarma, the process of detoxification and rejuvenation, can be correlated with modern understanding of metabolic processes and the body's natural cleansing mechanisms. While the specific techniques employed in Panchakarma differ from conventional detoxification methods, the underlying principle – that removing accumulated toxins can improve overall health and well-being – aligns with modern science's understanding of the body's ability to cleanse itself and the negative impact of toxins. The methods involved in Panchakarma, such as herbal enemas (Basti), oil massage (Abhyanga), and therapeutic sweating (Swedana), while traditional, might benefit from future research into the exact mechanisms by which they achieve their therapeutic effects.

The integration of Ayurveda and modern science is not about replacing one with the other; rather, it's about building a bridge between ancient wisdom and contemporary knowledge. It's about leveraging the strengths of both systems to create a more holistic and effective approach to healthcare. Ayurveda offers a personalized, preventative approach that addresses the root cause of imbalances, while modern science provides the tools to understand the underlying physiological and biochemical mechanisms.

This integration allows for a more nuanced understanding of health and disease. Modern diagnostic tools can help identify specific imbalances, while Ayurvedic principles can offer personalized strategies for restoring equilibrium. For instance, modern blood tests can reveal specific deficiencies, while Ayurvedic dietary and lifestyle recommendations can address these deficiencies naturally. Similarly, modern imaging techniques can identify structural abnormalities, while Ayurvedic treatments can support healing and promote overall well-being.

However, it is crucial to approach this integration with a critical and informed perspective. While modern science is constantly validating aspects of Ayurveda, rigorous scientific research is still needed to fully understand the mechanisms behind many traditional practices. It is essential to consult qualified and experienced practitioners of both Ayurvedic and modern medicine to ensure a safe and effective integration of both systems. The combined expertise offers a holistic and personalized approach to healing and well-being, creating a synergistic partnership that enhances both systems' effectiveness. This collaborative approach respects the validity of both ancient wisdom and modern scientific investigation, ultimately leading to a more comprehensive and effective approach to health and wellness.

The Role of the Panchamahabhutas Five Elements

Ayurveda views the universe and everything within it—including the human body—as being composed of five fundamental elements, known as the Panchamahabhutas: Akasha (ether), Vayu (air), Agni (fire), Jala (water), and Prithvi (earth). These elements aren't the same as the elements studied in Western chemistry; rather, they represent fundamental principles or qualities that manifest in different ways. Understanding these elements is crucial to grasping the Ayurvedic perspective on health and well-being because they form the basis of the three doshas (Vata, Pitta, and Kapha), which we explored in the previous chapter, and their interactions within the body.

Akasha, or ether, is the subtlest of the five elements. It represents space, the capacity for expansion, and the potential for all other elements to exist. Think of it as the void that allows for everything else to take form. In the body, Akasha is associated with the spaces within our body—the cavities like the lungs, stomach, and intestines. A healthy Akasha manifests as a sense of spaciousness, both physically and mentally, a feeling of freedom from constriction or
limitation. An imbalance can lead to feelings of being overwhelmed, claustrophobic, or lacking in clarity.

Vayu, or air, is characterized by movement, dynamism, and the principle of change. It represents the breath, circulation, and nervous system's function. In the body, Vayu governs functions like respiration, nerve impulses, and the circulation of blood and other fluids. A balanced Vayu manifests as lightness, agility, clarity of mind, and the ability to adapt to change. An excess of Vayu might lead to anxiety, nervousness, insomnia, or digestive issues characterized by gas and bloating. Conversely, a deficiency might manifest as lethargy, stiffness, and constipation.

Agni, or fire, embodies transformation, metabolism, and digestion. It's not just about the literal fire in our digestive tract; it's the transformative power that breaks down food, converts it into energy, and eliminates waste. Agni is the metabolic fire that sustains life. A strong Agni leads to efficient digestion, regular elimination, and a robust immune system. Conversely, a weak Agni can result in indigestion, bloating, weight gain, low energy levels, and a weakened immune response. It's important to note that Agni isn't confined to the digestive tract; it governs all transformative processes within the body, including the breakdown of toxins and the creation of new cells.

Jala, or water, represents fluidity, lubrication, and nourishment. It's the element that provides cohesion and balance to the body. In the body, Jala governs the fluids—blood, lymph, saliva, and other bodily fluids. A balanced Jala supports healthy hydration, lubrication of joints, and the smooth functioning of all bodily systems. An imbalance might manifest as dryness, dehydration, skin problems, constipation, or emotional rigidity.

Prithvi, or earth, represents stability, structure, and grounding. It's the element that gives form and substance to the body. In the body, Prithvi governs the tissues—bones, muscles, skin, and fat. A balanced Prithvi provides a sense of stability, strength, and grounding. Imbalances might present as weakness, fatigue, skin issues, weight changes, and lack of stability in physical or emotional life.

The interplay between these five elements is dynamic and constantly shifting. No element exists in isolation; they interact and influence each other, creating a complex and interconnected system. For example, the transformation of food (Agni) requires the movement of air (Vayu) and fluids (Jala) to transport nutrients to the tissues (Prithvi), all within the space (Akasha) of the body.

Understanding the Panchamahabhutas is crucial for understanding your own individual constitution, or Prakriti. Your Prakriti is determined by the unique balance of these five elements within you at the time of your birth. This balance influences your physical characteristics, personality traits, and susceptibility to certain diseases. While your Prakriti remains relatively constant throughout your life, your Vikriti (imbalance) can change depending on your lifestyle choices, environmental factors, and emotional state. Ayurveda aims to restore balance between these elements by addressing the Vikriti through dietary modifications, lifestyle changes, and herbal remedies.

The connection between the Panchamahabhutas and the three doshas is direct and fundamental. Each dosha is characterized by a unique combination of the five elements:

Vata:
This dosha is primarily composed of Akasha (ether) and Vayu (air). This explains its characteristics of movement, dryness, lightness, and change. The predominance of air accounts for the quick, often erratic nature of Vata, whereas the presence of ether allows for flexibility and adaptability. However, this can also lead to an excess of movement, resulting in anxiety, insomnia, and digestive irregularities if not properly balanced.

Pitta:
This dosha is predominantly composed of Agni (fire) and Jala (water). The fiery nature of Pitta is responsible for its transformative power, its intensity, and its sharp intellect. The presence of water provides fluidity, but also indicates a potential for imbalance leading to inflammation, anger, and

digestive issues associated with excess heat. Understanding this elemental composition helps to explain Pitta's connection to digestion, metabolism, and transformation.

Kapha:
This dosha is composed primarily of Prithvi (earth) and Jala (water). The earthy nature of Kapha lends itself to stability, structure, and grounding. The presence of water provides lubrication, support, and nourishment. This explains Kapha's connection to the physical structure of the body, its nurturing qualities, and its tendency towards stability, but also potential susceptibility to stagnation, excess weight, and sluggishness if the balance is disturbed.

The Panchamahabhutas also play a significant role in seasonal variations and how we adapt our lifestyle and diet to maintain balance. Each season is dominated by certain elements, influencing the doshas and requiring adjustments to our routines to maintain equilibrium. For instance, the dry, windy nature of autumn emphasizes Vata, while the intense heat of summer accentuates Pitta. Understanding this seasonal influence, combined with knowledge of your individual dosha, helps to create a personalized Ayurvedic lifestyle that adapts to the fluctuating energies throughout the year.

The principles of the Panchamahabhutas extend beyond the human body. They are essential in understanding the world around us and how our internal environment interacts with external influences. Ayurveda utilizes this knowledge to understand the effect of environmental factors on health, such as climate, diet, and lifestyle choices, and to tailor treatments and recommendations to promote optimal balance within each individual. The goal isn't simply to eliminate imbalance but to understand the elemental interplay and restore harmony.

For example, a person with a Vata imbalance might experience dryness and increased nervous activity. An Ayurvedic approach might suggest increasing the intake of grounding foods rich in earth elements (such as root vegetables) and reducing exposure to windy or cold environments. Similarly, a person with a Pitta imbalance might experience excessive heat and inflammation. In such a case, Ayurvedic recommendations would likely focus on cooling foods and activities, promoting a reduction of fiery Pitta. A Kapha imbalance, on the other hand, might necessitate increased movement and lighter, more easily digestible foods to counteract sluggishness and promote balance.

The ancient wisdom encoded within the Panchamahabhutas offers a profound and holistic understanding of health and well-being. By recognizing the interconnectedness of the five elements within ourselves and the world around us, we can develop a deeper appreciation of the subtle forces that shape our health and experience a more balanced and fulfilling life. This understanding forms the cornerstone of Ayurvedic diagnosis and treatment, guiding practitioners in identifying imbalances and creating personalized strategies to restore harmony within the individual's unique constitution. The five elements are not simply abstract concepts; they are tangible forces that shape our existence, offering a roadmap to holistic well-being. Recognizing and working with these elements, rather than against them, is a key step toward achieving optimal health in an Ayurvedic context.

Setting Your Intentions for an Ayurvedic Journey

Embarking on an Ayurvedic journey is a commitment to holistic well-being, a path of self-discovery and mindful living. It's not a quick fix or a fad diet; rather, it's a transformative process that requires patience, self-compassion, and a willingness to embrace change at your own pace. Setting realistic intentions is paramount to success. Avoid the temptation to overhaul your entire life overnight. Instead, focus on integrating Ayurvedic principles gradually and sustainably, building a foundation of healthy habits that you can maintain long-term.

One of the most common pitfalls is setting overly ambitious goals. Aspiring to completely change your diet, sleep schedule, and exercise routine all at once is a recipe for burnout and frustration. This approach often leads to feelings of overwhelm and ultimately, abandonment of the Ayurvedic path. Remember, the journey is just as important as the destination. Celebrate small victories and acknowledge that setbacks are a natural part of the process. They provide valuable learning opportunities and a chance to refine your approach.

Start by identifying one or two areas where you'd like to focus your efforts. Perhaps you'd like to improve your sleep hygiene, incorporate more fresh fruits and vegetables into your diet, or establish a regular meditation practice. Choose areas that resonate with you and that you feel confident you can incorporate into your daily routine without causing undue stress. This focused approach will allow you to build momentum and experience tangible results, fueling your motivation and commitment to continue the journey.

For example, let's say your primary goal is to improve your digestion. Instead of completely overhauling your diet immediately, begin by incorporating one or two simple changes. You could start by drinking a warm cup of water with lemon first thing in the morning to stimulate digestion or by practicing mindful eating, paying close attention to the taste, texture, and aroma of your food. These small, manageable steps will pave the way for larger dietary changes later on, as your awareness and understanding of your body's needs deepen.

Another crucial aspect of setting intentions is aligning them with your unique doshic constitution. As discussed previously, understanding your predominant dosha—Vata, Pitta, or Kapha—is fundamental to creating a personalized Ayurvedic plan that caters to your individual needs and temperament. For instance, if you have a predominantly Vata constitution, characterized by its airy and mobile nature, you might choose to focus on grounding practices such as grounding yoga poses, regular massage with warm sesame oil (Abhyanga), and incorporating warming foods and spices into your diet to help stabilize your Vata energy.

Conversely, if your predominant dosha is Pitta, known for its fiery and transformative nature, you might prioritize cooling practices such as regular meditation, spending time in nature, and consuming cooling foods and drinks. This might include incorporating foods rich in cucumber, coconut water, and mint into your daily meal plan.

For those with a Kapha constitution, which is characterized by its earthy and stable nature, the focus might be on incorporating stimulating activities into their daily routine, such as brisk walks, light exercise, and a diet that is lighter and less oily. These individuals might benefit from incorporating spices like ginger and black pepper to help ignite their digestive fire. Tailoring your intentions to your specific dosha ensures that your efforts are aligned with your unique constitution, leading to more effective and sustainable results.

Beyond diet and exercise, setting intentions also extends to other crucial aspects of Ayurvedic well-being, such as sleep, stress management, and mindful self-care. Aim to establish a regular sleep schedule, aiming for 7-8 hours of quality sleep each night. Explore different stress-reduction techniques, such as yoga, meditation, or spending time in nature. Prioritize self-care activities that nourish your mind, body, and spirit, such as taking a warm bath, listening to soothing music, or engaging in activities that bring you joy and relaxation. These practices, when integrated into your daily routine, can contribute to a more harmonious and balanced life.

It's essential to remember that Ayurveda is not just about following a set of rules; it's a journey of self-discovery and a lifelong commitment to holistic well-being. Setting intentions should be an ongoing process, one that evolves as you deepen your understanding of your body and its unique needs. Regularly review and adjust your goals based on your progress, challenges, and shifting priorities. This flexibility is essential for maintaining long-term adherence and ensuring that your Ayurvedic practices remain a source of joy and vitality rather than a burden.

Moreover, setting intentions shouldn't be a solitary endeavor. Consider seeking support from a qualified Ayurvedic practitioner or joining a community of like-minded individuals who are also on an Ayurvedic journey. Sharing your experiences, challenges, and triumphs with others can provide invaluable support, encouragement, and motivation. Connecting with a community can create a sense of belonging and camaraderie, strengthening your commitment to the path and offering valuable resources and insights.

Ayurveda is a deeply personalized system. What works for one person may not work for another. Therefore, it's vital to listen to your body and trust your intuition. Pay attention to how your body responds to different practices and adjust your intentions accordingly. If something doesn't feel right, don't force it. Experiment with different approaches and find what resonates with you and brings you a sense of balance and well-being.

Your intentions should also be infused with compassion and self-acceptance. Embrace imperfection and understand that setbacks are a natural part of the process. Don't let occasional lapses derail your progress. Instead, acknowledge them, learn from them, and gently guide yourself back onto the path. Self-compassion is crucial for maintaining a positive and sustainable relationship with your Ayurvedic practices.

Finally, remember that the ultimate goal of Ayurveda is not just physical health, but holistic well-being, encompassing physical, mental, and spiritual dimensions. Setting intentions that encompass all aspects of your life will ensure that your Ayurvedic journey is truly transformative and leads to a more fulfilling and balanced existence. Consider incorporating intentions that foster inner peace, cultivate gratitude, and strengthen your connection to your inner self. These inner aspects are just as crucial as physical health in creating a life filled with joy, purpose, and vitality. By taking a holistic approach to setting intentions, you are laying a strong foundation for a truly rewarding and sustainable Ayurvedic journey. This path of self-discovery and mindful living will guide you towards a state of optimal well-being, allowing you to thrive in every aspect of your life.

Physical and Mental Characteristics

Understanding the three doshas—Vata, Pitta, and Kapha—is foundational to Ayurvedic practice. Each dosha represents a unique combination of the five elements (ether, air, fire, water, and earth) and governs specific physiological and psychological functions within the body. By understanding your predominant dosha and its characteristics, you can gain valuable insights into your constitution, tendencies, and potential imbalances. This understanding empowers you to make informed choices about your lifestyle, diet, and self-care practices to maintain optimal health and well-being.

Let's delve into a detailed examination of the physical and mental characteristics associated with each dosha. Remember, most individuals possess a combination of doshas, with one typically being more dominant. This assessment aims to help you identify your primary dosha and understand its influence on your life.

Vata Dosha: The Air and Ether Principle

Vata, characterized by the elements of air and ether, is associated with movement, change, and creativity. Individuals with a predominant Vata dosha often exhibit a lean, agile physique. Their bodies may appear somewhat delicate, and they might experience dryness of skin and hair. Their energy levels can fluctuate dramatically, often feeling energized and exhilarated one moment, and exhausted and depleted the next. Sleep can be elusive, and they may experience insomnia or restless sleep.

Mentally, Vata individuals are often quick-witted, imaginative, and adaptable. Their minds are constantly in motion, leading to creativity and innovation but also potential anxiety and nervousness. They are prone to scattered thoughts and may struggle with focus and concentration. They are often enthusiastic and energetic but can be easily overwhelmed by stress or change. Their emotions can shift rapidly, reflecting the dynamic nature of the Vata dosha. Symptoms of Vata imbalance often include constipation, dry skin, anxiety, insomnia, and cold extremities.

Examples of Vata Characteristics:

Physical:
Thin build, dry skin and hair, cold hands and feet, irregular digestion, frequent gas, light sleep, prone to constipation, quick movements, and sometimes easily bruised.

Mental:
Creative, imaginative, quick-witted, adaptable, enthusiastic, easily distracted, prone to anxiety, nervousness, and fear. Can experience periods of intense energy followed by exhaustion.

Pitta Dosha: The Fire and Water Principle

Pitta, governed by the elements of fire and water, represents transformation, metabolism, and digestion. Individuals with a predominantly Pitta constitution often have a medium build and a strong, athletic physique. Their skin is usually warm and possibly oily, with a tendency toward redness or irritation. They possess a strong digestive system and often have a robust appetite. They are generally energetic and have a strong drive to achieve their goals.

Mentally, Pitta individuals are sharp, intelligent, and focused. They are ambitious, assertive, and possess a strong sense of self. They are excellent leaders and often excel in competitive environments. However, their intense nature can also lead to irritability, impatience, and anger. They are detail-oriented and meticulous, often perfectionistic in their approach to tasks. Symptoms of Pitta imbalance can manifest as heartburn, indigestion, ulcers, skin rashes, inflammation, and anger.

Examples of Pitta Characteristics:

Physical:
Medium build, warm body temperature, oily skin, reddish complexion, strong digestive system, strong appetite, and can easily become overheated.
Mental:
Intelligent, ambitious, focused, assertive, decisive, confident, can be impatient, irritable, easily angered, and perfectionistic.

Kapha Dosha: The Earth and Water Principle

Kapha, dominated by the elements of earth and water, embodies stability, structure, and grounding. Individuals with a predominant Kapha dosha often have a larger, more robust physique. Their skin is generally soft, smooth, and moist. They are usually slow-paced and steady in their movements and actions. They tend to have a stable weight and strong immunity. They often enjoy sleeping long and deeply.

Mentally, Kapha individuals are calm, patient, and compassionate. They are loyal, loving, and grounded. They possess a strong sense of empathy and are often nurturing and supportive. However, their stable nature can also make them resistant to change and prone to complacency or inertia. They often enjoy routine and prefer a predictable lifestyle. Symptoms of Kapha imbalance may include weight gain, lethargy, water retention, congestion, and sluggishness.

Examples of Kapha Characteristics:

Physical:
Strong build, soft, moist skin, slower metabolism, often heavier build, strong immunity, and tends to have a slower pace of life.

Mental:
Calm, patient, compassionate, loving, supportive, loyal, stable, can be resistant to change, and prone to complacency or inertia.

Beyond the Basics: Understanding Doshic Combinations

It's crucial to remember that most individuals don't perfectly fit into just one doshic category. Instead, they usually have a combination of doshas, with one being dominant and others present in lesser amounts. For example, someone might be primarily Pitta with secondary Vata characteristics. This means they might share the ambitious nature of Pitta but also experience some of the anxiety and scattered energy of Vata. Understanding these combinations allows for a more nuanced and personalized approach to Ayurvedic self-care.

Identifying Your Imbalances:

Recognizing imbalances within your dosha is essential for maintaining optimal health. These imbalances, also known as
Vikriti
, arise when the elements within your constitution are out of harmony. Paying attention to your physical and mental sensations, energy levels, and emotional states can offer valuable clues about potential imbalances. For instance, a Vata individual experiencing increased anxiety and insomnia might be experiencing a Vata aggravation. Similarly, a Pitta individual with frequent heartburn and anger issues may be exhibiting signs of Pitta imbalance. A Kapha individual struggling with weight gain and lethargy may indicate a Kapha imbalance. The next section will delve

into specific strategies for recognizing and addressing these imbalances. By understanding your dosha and its potential imbalances, you can proactively adjust your lifestyle and diet to maintain balance and well-being. The goal is not to rigidly adhere to a specific dosha type, but to use this understanding as a guide to nourish and support your unique constitution. This involves making conscious choices regarding diet, exercise, and lifestyle that are in harmony with your individual needs.

A Visual Guide to SelfIdentification

The journey to understanding your Ayurvedic constitution begins with self-reflection. While the descriptions of Vata, Pitta, and Kapha offer a solid foundation, individual expressions are nuanced and unique. The Dosha Wheel, presented here, provides a visual framework to aid your self-identification process. This isn't a definitive test; rather, it's a tool to guide your introspection and facilitate a deeper understanding of your own energetic blueprint.

Imagine the Dosha Wheel as a three-part circle, each section representing one of the three doshas: Vata, Pitta, and Kapha. Within each section, you'll find a series of characteristics related to physical attributes, mental and emotional tendencies, and digestive patterns. As you consider each characteristic, assess how strongly it resonates with your personal experience. Do you strongly identify with several traits within one section? Or do you find yourself recognizing aspects of multiple doshas? This is perfectly normal; most individuals exhibit a combination of doshic traits, with one or two typically being more dominant.

Let's explore each segment of the Dosha Wheel in detail. Begin by focusing on the
physical
characteristics. Consider your body type: are you lean and wiry (Vata), medium build and muscular (Pitta), or larger and more robust (Kapha)?
This offers a preliminary indication, but isn't solely determinative. Examine your skin: is it dry and prone to wrinkles (Vata), warm and sometimes oily with freckles or blemishes (Pitta), or soft, smooth, and moist (Kapha)? The quality of your hair offers further clues: thin, dry, and perhaps slightly brittle (Vata), fine or medium texture (Pitta), or thick, lustrous, and possibly oily (Kapha). Think about

your nails – are they brittle and easily broken (Vata), strong but may have ridges (Pitta), or strong, thick, and pink (Kapha)?

Beyond the obvious, delve into the subtler aspects of physicality. Consider your energy levels. Does your energy fluctuate wildly, with periods of intense activity followed by exhaustion (Vata)? Or is your energy steady and consistent throughout the day (Pitta or Kapha)? Do you find yourself feeling easily fatigued (Kapha), or do you have a naturally high energy level (Vata and Pitta)? Consider your digestion: is your appetite variable and sometimes erratic (Vata), strong and with a tendency toward heat and acidity (Pitta), or generally good but prone to sluggishness (Kapha)? Your bowel movements provide further insights: irregular and often accompanied by gas (Vata), often loose or potentially leading to diarrhea (Pitta), or regular but potentially constipated (Kapha). Your sleep patterns also tell a story; is it often disrupted and light (Vata), generally sound but maybe interrupted by hot flashes or nightmares (Pitta), or long and restful, sometimes even excessively so (Kapha)? Observe your tolerance for cold and heat; do you feel the cold intensely (Vata), prefer moderate temperatures (Pitta), and easily overheat (Kapha)?

Moving beyond the physical realm, the Dosha Wheel guides you into the mental and emotional landscape. Consider your mental activity. Are you prone to scattered thoughts and anxieties (Vata), focused and driven, potentially even prone to irritability (Pitta), or calm and thoughtful, perhaps sometimes prone to inertia (Kapha)? Examine your emotional patterns: Are you highly sensitive and prone to emotional fluctuations (Vata), easily angered or frustrated (Pitta), or generally calm and stable but susceptible to clinginess or possessiveness (Kapha)? Assess your creativity and adaptability: are you inventive and quick to adapt (Vata), systematic and ambitious, possessing a strong sense of direction (Pitta), or methodical and loyal, preferring routine and stability (Kapha)? Consider your communication style: Do you tend to speak rapidly and perhaps change topics frequently (Vata)? Are you direct and to-the-point, even assertive (Pitta)? Or are you calm, slow to speak, but deeply thoughtful (Kapha)?

Your cognitive style also offers clues. Are you quick-witted and insightful but also prone to mental exhaustion (Vata)? Do you possess a sharp intellect and the capacity for focused concentration (Pitta)? Or is your thinking thoughtful, measured, and grounded in practical considerations (Kapha)? Finally, consider your approach to life; are you impulsive and adaptable, easily embracing change (Vata)? Are you goal-oriented, efficient, and decisive (Pitta)? Or are you methodical, steady, and patient, prioritizing consistency (Kapha)?

By thoughtfully considering these aspects of your physical and mental being, you'll start to notice patterns emerging. You might find a strong resonance within one section of the Dosha Wheel, indicating a predominance of a specific dosha. Alternatively, you may find a more balanced distribution, suggesting a blend of doshas with one or two being more dominant. Remember, this is not a rigid categorization; rather, it's a dynamic interplay of energies that shifts and evolves throughout your life, influenced by factors such as season, diet, stress, and lifestyle choices.

Let's illustrate this with some examples. Imagine someone who describes themselves as constantly busy, with racing thoughts, a tendency towards anxiety, and a body that is thin and easily chilled. They experience irregular sleep, digestive disturbances, and rapid speech. This individual would likely identify strongly with the Vata characteristics on the Dosha

Wheel. Conversely, someone who describes themselves as having strong digestive fire, a propensity for sharp focus and ambition, and a medium build with warm skin would find more resonance with the Pitta qualities. This person might also describe a tendency towards being opinionated and decisive. Finally, someone with a calm disposition, a strong, robust build, and a tendency toward weight gain, coupled with a slow metabolism and a love for routine, would align strongly with the Kapha characteristics on the Dosha Wheel.

However, remember that these are simplified examples. A person might have predominantly Pitta characteristics, but exhibit some Kapha tendencies in their emotional stability or Vata tendencies in their occasional bursts of creative energy. The Dosha Wheel helps illuminate these nuances, guiding you towards a deeper understanding of your unique constitution. The key is to avoid labeling yourself rigidly; rather, use this understanding as a roadmap for creating a lifestyle that supports your inherent balance and well-being. The Dosha Wheel is just the beginning of a journey – a journey of self-discovery that empowers you to live a more harmonious and fulfilling life in accordance with your natural constitution. In subsequent chapters, we will delve deeper into each dosha, offering personalized strategies for maintaining balance and addressing imbalances.

This understanding of your dosha is not a static label but a dynamic guide that evolves with time, season, and lifestyle choices. Understanding your inherent doshic constitution acts as a foundation for building a personalized approach to wellness. Your dosha is not a fixed characteristic but a living energy that is constantly interacting with your environment and experiences. As you journey through life, you will learn to recognize how external factors influence your dosha, helping you make adjustments in your diet, lifestyle, and daily routine to maintain optimal well-being. The process of self-identification is continuous; it's an ongoing dialogue with your body and mind, refining your understanding and strengthening your capacity to live in harmony with your unique constitution.

As you work with the Dosha Wheel, remember that self-observation is key. Pay attention to your body's signals—your energy levels, digestive patterns, sleep quality, and emotional responses. These clues will help you refine your understanding of your dosha and guide your decisions regarding diet, exercise, and lifestyle choices. This isn't about achieving perfection but about striving for balance. Ayurveda is a journey, not a destination, and each step you take towards self-understanding brings you closer to a healthier, happier, and more balanced life. The Dosha Wheel is simply a valuable tool to help you begin this transformative journey. Embrace the process, celebrate your unique constitution, and embark on the path towards optimal well-being.

Understanding Your Doshic Imbalances

Understanding your dosha is the first step towards achieving optimal health and well-being within the framework of Ayurveda. However, the journey doesn't end with identification. Life's stresses, dietary indiscretions, and seasonal changes can all contribute to doshic imbalances, leading to various physical and mental health concerns. Recognizing these imbalances is crucial to restoring equilibrium.

Let's delve into the common imbalances associated with each dosha and explore practical strategies to address them.

Vata Imbalance:
Vata dosha, characterized by air and ether, governs movement and creativity. When Vata is imbalanced, it often manifests as dryness, coldness, and excessive movement. Think of a whirlwind – chaotic and unpredictable. Symptoms of Vata imbalance can range from mild discomfort to severe health problems. Common indicators include:

Digestive issues:
Constipation, bloating, gas, irregular bowel movements, and a feeling of dryness in the digestive tract are frequent signs. The dryness can extend to the skin, leading to cracked lips and dry skin. The digestive system's efficiency is compromised, resulting in poor nutrient absorption and potential weight loss.

Nervous system disturbances:
Anxiety, insomnia, nervousness, tremors, and a scattered mind are common manifestations. This imbalance can make it difficult to focus, leading to reduced concentration and poor memory recall. The constant internal "churning" associated with Vata

imbalance often translates into restlessness and difficulty relaxing.

Musculoskeletal problems:
Joint pain, stiffness, and muscle spasms are frequently experienced. The dryness associated with Vata can affect the joints, leading to pain and reduced mobility. This can further lead to decreased physical activity and contribute to a vicious cycle of discomfort.

Other symptoms:
Cold intolerance, dry skin and hair, dizziness, palpitations, and a tendency towards fatigue can also be indicative of a Vata imbalance. The overall feeling is often one of instability and unease. The body feels vulnerable and easily depleted.

Addressing Vata Imbalance:
The key to balancing Vata lies in adopting a lifestyle that promotes grounding and stability.
This involves incorporating warming, moistening, and grounding elements into your daily routine.

Dietary Adjustments:
Include warming spices like ginger, cinnamon, and cardamom in your meals. Focus on warm, cooked foods rather than raw salads and cold drinks.
Incorporate nourishing foods like soups, stews, and cooked vegetables. Increase your intake of healthy fats such as ghee (clarified butter), olive oil, and avocado. Avoid dry, cold foods like ice cream, raw vegetables, and overly processed foods. Regularly consume warm herbal teas, like chamomile or ginger tea.

Lifestyle Modifications:
Establish a regular sleep schedule, ensuring you get adequate rest. Practice calming activities like yoga, meditation, or pranayama (breathing exercises). Create a sense of routine and predictability in your daily life to reduce anxiety. Avoid overexertion and prioritize
relaxation. Engage in activities that bring you joy and help you feel grounded, such as spending time in nature. Massage

with warm sesame oil can also help to soothe and nourish the tissues, reducing dryness.

Herbal Remedies:
Consult with an Ayurvedic practitioner to explore herbal remedies that can help to pacify Vata, such as Ashwagandha, Shatavari, and Jatamansi. These herbs possess calming and balancing properties that can be
beneficial in restoring equilibrium.

Pitta Imbalance:
Pitta, governed by fire and water,
represents transformation and metabolism. When Pitta is out of balance, it often leads to excessive heat, inflammation, and acidity. Think of a raging fire – intense and potentially destructive. Symptoms of Pitta imbalance can vary from mild discomfort to serious health problems.

Digestive issues:
Heartburn, acid reflux, gastritis, ulcers, and diarrhea are commonly associated with Pitta imbalances.
The increased heat and acidity can disrupt the delicate balance of the digestive system, leading to various problems.

Skin problems:
Acne, rashes, boils, and skin inflammation are common manifestations of excessive Pitta. The increased heat and inflammation can manifest directly on the skin, causing irritation and discomfort.

Emotional disturbances:
Irritability, anger, frustration, and impatience are often linked to Pitta imbalances. The fiery nature of Pitta when unbalanced can lead to impulsive actions and heightened emotional reactions.

Other symptoms:
Fever, headaches, inflammation,
excessive sweating, and a tendency towards ulcers are also indicative of Pitta imbalances. This often creates a feeling of internal heat and pressure.

Addressing Pitta Imbalance:
The strategy for balancing Pitta involves cooling, soothing, and calming the body and mind.

Dietary Adjustments:
Focus on cooling foods such as cucumbers, spinach, coconut, and lettuce. Incorporate sweet,

bitter, and astringent tastes into your diet. Reduce your consumption of spicy, hot, and sour foods. Avoid excessive caffeine and alcohol. Choose hydrating fruits like watermelon and berries.

Lifestyle Modifications:
Prioritize rest and relaxation. Avoid strenuous exercise during the hottest parts of the day.
Practice calming activities such as yoga, meditation, and spending time in nature, particularly near water. Create a calm and peaceful environment. Avoid overworking and stress. Engage in calming activities to soothe the mind.

Herbal Remedies:
Consult with an Ayurvedic practitioner to explore herbs like Guduchi (Tinospora cordifolia) and Amalaki (Emblica officinalis), known for their cooling and balancing properties. These herbs can help to restore equilibrium and reduce inflammation.

Kapha Imbalance:
Kapha, composed of water and earth, represents structure, stability, and grounding. When Kapha is imbalanced, it can manifest as sluggishness, heaviness, and stagnation. Think of a stagnant swamp – slow, heavy, and prone to buildup. Symptoms of Kapha imbalance can range from mild lethargy to more serious health conditions.

Digestive issues:
Bloating, sluggish digestion, constipation, increased mucus production, and water retention are
common symptoms. Kapha's tendency toward heaviness can directly impact the digestive system, leading to reduced efficiency.

Respiratory issues:
Increased mucus production,
congestion, and respiratory infections are frequently observed. The heavy, damp nature of Kapha can clog the respiratory passages.

Emotional disturbances:
Apathy, depression, clinginess, and attachment issues can be

associated with an imbalanced Kapha. The sluggishness of an imbalanced Kapha can affect the emotional realm, creating feelings of inertia and stagnation.

Other symptoms:
Weight gain, edema (swelling), fatigue, lethargy, and a tendency towards colds and flu are also symptoms. This can result in a feeling of physical heaviness and a lack of energy.

Addressing Kapha Imbalance:
The approach to balancing Kapha focuses on stimulating the body's natural processes and promoting lightness and movement.

Dietary Adjustments:
Incorporate pungent, bitter, and astringent tastes into your diet. Focus on lighter, easily digestible foods. Increase your intake of spices like ginger, cumin, and black pepper. Reduce your consumption of heavy, greasy, and sweet foods. Choose warm, cooked foods over cold, heavy dishes.

Lifestyle Modifications:
Engage in regular physical activity to increase circulation and metabolism. Incorporate dynamic yoga poses and cardio exercises. Avoid prolonged periods of inactivity or rest. Practice pranayama (breathing exercises) to improve lung function and enhance energy levels. Keep your environment clean and organized.

Herbal Remedies:
Consult with an Ayurvedic practitioner to explore herbs such as Pippali (long pepper) and Ginger, which are known for their warming and stimulating properties. These can help to reduce sluggishness and increase metabolic activity.

It is crucial to remember that these are general guidelines. Individual experiences may vary. The best approach to managing doshic imbalances is to work with a qualified Ayurvedic practitioner who can create a personalized plan tailored to your unique constitution and current health status. Ayurveda is a holistic system, and addressing imbalances requires a comprehensive approach that considers diet, lifestyle, and mental well-being. The journey towards balance is a personal one, and with consistent effort and self-awareness, you can achieve optimal health and well-being. Remember that small, sustainable changes can make a significant difference over time. Embrace the process, be patient with yourself, and enjoy the journey towards a healthier and more balanced you.

Initial Steps

Now that you've discovered your predominant dosha, let's embark on a journey towards cultivating balance and well-being through practical lifestyle adjustments. Remember, Ayurveda is a holistic system; these recommendations are starting points, not rigid rules. Listen to your body, observe its responses, and adjust accordingly. A qualified Ayurvedic practitioner can provide personalized guidance based on your unique constitution and current health status.

Vata Dosha: Nurturing Stability and Grounding

Individuals with a predominantly Vata constitution often experience dryness, lightness, and coolness. Their energy can be erratic, leading to anxiety, insomnia, and digestive issues. The key to balancing Vata is to incorporate practices that promote grounding, stability, and warmth.

Dietary Recommendations:
Focus on warm, cooked foods with grounding qualities. Include plenty of warming spices like ginger, cinnamon, and cardamom in your meals.
Embrace foods rich in healthy fats, such as ghee (clarified butter), avocado, and nuts. Regularly consume soups and stews, as well as root vegetables like sweet potatoes and carrots. Avoid raw salads and cold drinks, opting instead for warm herbal teas. Incorporate grounding grains like quinoa and brown rice into your diet. Prioritize foods that are easily digestible to avoid exacerbating Vata's tendency towards digestive irregularities. Consider incorporating warming oils into your cooking like coconut oil.

Lifestyle Adjustments:
Establish a consistent daily routine (Dinacharya). Prioritize regular sleep, aiming for 7-8 hours

of uninterrupted rest. Create a calming bedtime routine that includes warm baths, gentle massage with sesame oil (Abhyanga), and meditation. Minimize stress through practices like yoga, pranayama (breathing exercises), and meditation. Avoid overstimulation from caffeine, excessive travel, or erratic schedules. Schedule regular massage therapy for lubrication and grounding the body. Incorporate grounding activities such as spending time in nature, listening to calming music, and engaging in creative pursuits. Avoid exposure to harsh weather conditions, and dress warmly. Avoid excessive physical activity that exhausts the nervous system.

Pitta Dosha: Cooling and Calming the Fiery Energy

Individuals with a predominantly Pitta constitution are often characterized by a fiery, intense, and transformative energy. They might experience anger, irritability, heartburn, and inflammation. The goal is to cool down this fiery energy and promote a sense of calm and balance.

Dietary Recommendations:
Prioritize cooling foods like cucumbers, lettuce, coconut water, and yogurt. Incorporate sweet and bitter tastes, like berries and leafy greens, into your diet. Avoid excessive spicy, sour, and pungent foods that can further increase Pitta. Limit caffeine and alcohol, which can exacerbate Pitta's fiery nature. Opt for lighter meals that are easy to digest. Introduce foods rich in fiber to support healthy bowel movements and reduce Pitta's
tendency towards heat and inflammation. Regularly consume foods like aloe vera for its cooling properties.

Lifestyle Adjustments:
Cultivate a calming atmosphere in your home and work environment. Practice stress-reducing techniques like meditation, deep breathing exercises, and gentle yoga. Avoid excessive heat, either from the

environment or intense physical activity. Schedule regular breaks to prevent burnout. Incorporate cooling activities such as swimming, spending time near water bodies, or taking cool showers. Prioritize regular sleep and avoid working late into the night. Ensure your workplace is well-ventilated and not overly heated. Manage your emotions effectively through mindfulness practices. Seek opportunities to cool down through relaxation techniques.

Kapha Dosha: Stimulating Energy and Lightness

Individuals with a predominantly Kapha constitution are often characterized by grounded stability, strength, and resilience. They may experience sluggishness, weight gain, and respiratory congestion. Balancing Kapha requires stimulating the body's energy and promoting lightness.

Dietary Recommendations:
Favor light, easily digestible foods such as whole grains, legumes, and fresh vegetables. Reduce the intake of heavy, oily, and sweet foods.
Incorporate pungent and bitter tastes, which help to stimulate digestion and reduce Kapha. Spices such as ginger, turmeric, and black pepper can assist in stimulating the digestive fire (agni). Consume foods that are warm and dry instead of cold and moist. Avoid excessive dairy products and sweets. Encourage light snacks to keep energy levels steady and reduce overeating. Favor warming spices to increase metabolic rate. Increase the consumption of cruciferous vegetables known for their cleansing properties.

Lifestyle Adjustments:
Increase physical activity through brisk walking, jogging, or cycling. Practice energizing yoga styles such as Vinyasa or Ashtanga. Engage in activities that boost circulation and metabolic processes. Prioritize early mornings and maintain a disciplined routine, avoiding
oversleeping. Ensure adequate ventilation in your living

space. Avoid overindulgence in sleep and sensual pleasures, as these can further increase Kapha. Spend time outdoors to get fresh air and sunshine. Regularly practice pranayama (breathing exercises) to enhance lung capacity and boost energy levels. Consider incorporating activities that promote mindfulness and alertness. Maintain an organized environment to reduce the tendency towards stagnation. Engage in light stretching or mobility exercises, rather than strenuous physical activity.

Additional Considerations:

Beyond these dosha-specific recommendations, there are several universal Ayurvedic principles that promote overall well-being. These include:

Dinacharya (Daily Routine):
Establishing a consistent daily routine is crucial for maintaining balance. This
includes waking early, practicing self-care, eating at regular intervals, and getting adequate sleep.

Ritucharya (Seasonal Adjustments):
Ayurveda emphasizes adapting to the changing seasons. Your diet and lifestyle should shift with the transitions to maintain harmony with nature.

Stress Management:
Chronic stress disrupts the doshas, so practicing stress reduction techniques like yoga, meditation, and spending time in nature is essential.

Proper Digestion (Agni):
Ayurveda places a strong
emphasis on healthy digestion. Eating mindfully, avoiding overeating, and using digestive aids as needed can significantly improve overall health.

Remember that these recommendations are a starting point for your Ayurvedic journey. The key is to listen to your body, observe its reactions, and make adjustments as needed. The goal is to create a personalized approach that supports your unique constitution and lifestyle. By integrating these principles into your daily life, you can begin to experience the transformative power of Ayurveda and move towards a more balanced and healthy existence. A qualified Ayurvedic practitioner can provide more personalized and in-depth guidance, ensuring your journey is tailored to your specific needs and circumstances. Consider seeking professional guidance for any underlying health conditions or when implementing significant lifestyle changes. The power of Ayurveda lies in its holistic approach; your journey towards well-being involves nurturing your physical, mental, and emotional states.

Addressing Seasonal Doshic Shifts and Adaptations

Ayurveda emphasizes the profound interconnectedness between our internal constitution (dosha) and the external environment. Just as the seasons shift and transform, so too does the balance within our bodies. Ignoring these seasonal fluctuations can lead to imbalances, manifesting as various physical and mental discomforts. Understanding and adapting to these seasonal doshic shifts is crucial for maintaining optimal health and well-being.

The Ayurvedic calendar divides the year into six seasons, each possessing unique energetic qualities that influence the three doshas – Vata, Pitta, and Kapha. By understanding these seasonal influences, we can proactively adjust our diet, lifestyle, and daily routines to mitigate potential imbalances and harness the beneficial aspects of each season.

Vata Season (Autumn and Early Winter):
Autumn and early winter are characterized by the dry, cold, and windy qualities of Vata. During this time, Vata dosha tends to become aggravated, leading to potential dryness of the skin and mucous membranes, constipation, anxiety, and insomnia. To counteract these effects, it's crucial to adopt a Vata-pacifying lifestyle. This involves incorporating warm, moist, and grounding elements into your daily routine.

Dietary adjustments are key. Focus on warm, cooked foods, rich in healthy fats and oils. Think hearty soups, stews, and warm porridges made with nourishing grains like barley or oats. Include plenty of warming spices like ginger, cinnamon, and cardamom in your cooking. These spices not only enhance the flavor but also help to generate internal heat and counteract the cold and dryness of the season. Increase your intake of grounding vegetables such as sweet potatoes, carrots, and beets. Nuts and seeds, particularly sesame seeds, are also excellent sources of healthy fats that support Vata balance. Minimize raw foods, salads, and cold drinks as they can further exacerbate Vata imbalances.

Beyond diet, incorporating grounding practices is vital. Regular massage with warm sesame oil (Abhyanga) can help to lubricate the tissues and soothe the nervous system. Gentle exercise such as yoga, focusing on slow, flowing movements, is preferable to rigorous workouts. Prioritize rest and relaxation. Establish a consistent sleep schedule, aiming for at least 7-8 hours of uninterrupted sleep. Meditation and pranayama (breathing exercises) can help to calm the mind and reduce anxiety. Create a warm and comforting environment in your home, using soft lighting, warm colors, and comfortable textiles to promote relaxation. Avoid exposure to harsh winds and cold temperatures whenever possible.

Pitta Season (Late Spring and Early Summer):
Late spring and early summer are characterized by the intense heat and fiery qualities of Pitta. During this time, Pitta dosha can become aggravated, leading to potential inflammation, heartburn, irritability, and skin rashes. A Pitta-pacifying lifestyle focuses on cooling, grounding practices that help to reduce heat and inflammation.

Dietary choices should emphasize cooling foods. Incorporate fresh fruits and vegetables, particularly those with a cooling effect, such as cucumbers, watermelon, and mint. Choose light, easily digestible foods, avoiding spicy and oily dishes. Opt for smaller, more frequent meals instead of large, heavy ones. Cooling beverages like coconut water or herbal infusions can help to quench thirst and reduce internal heat.

Minimize processed foods, caffeine, and alcohol, as these can aggravate Pitta. Regular hydration is crucial during this season.

Lifestyle adjustments include prioritizing rest and avoiding excessive sun exposure. Moderate exercise, such as swimming or gentle yoga, is beneficial, but avoid strenuous activity during the hottest parts of the day. Incorporate calming activities like spending time in nature under shady trees, listening to calming music, and engaging in creative pursuits. Minimize stress as much as possible; stress can easily exacerbate Pitta imbalances. Practice mindfulness and relaxation techniques to maintain a calm and balanced state of mind.

Kapha Season (Late Autumn and Winter):
Late autumn and winter are characterized by the heavy, slow, and cold qualities of Kapha. During this time, Kapha dosha can become sluggish, leading to potential weight gain, lethargy, and respiratory congestion. A Kapha-pacifying lifestyle focuses on stimulating, warming, and activating practices.

Dietary adjustments should emphasize light, easily digestible foods. Incorporate warming spices such as ginger, black pepper, and cumin to stimulate digestion. Reduce the consumption of heavy, rich foods, dairy products, and sweets. Choose foods with pungent and bitter tastes to stimulate the digestive fire and cleanse the system. Prioritize warming foods and drinks, such as herbal teas, and soups. Avoid excessive consumption of cold and heavy foods which can further aggravate Kapha. Light exercise is important during this period to counteract the sluggishness.

Lifestyle adjustments should focus on promoting circulation and energy levels. Regular exercise, such as brisk walking, yoga, or any activity that gets you moving, is important.

Engage in activities that stimulate the mind, such as reading, learning new skills, or engaging in stimulating conversations. Aim for a moderate amount of sunlight exposure to boost energy levels. Maintain a regular sleep schedule, while avoiding oversleeping. Ensure proper ventilation in your living spaces to promote good air circulation.

Transitional Periods:
The transition between seasons is particularly important. These periods often see an increase in doshic imbalances due to the changing environmental
conditions. It's crucial to pay attention to subtle shifts in your energy levels and physical sensations during these times and make appropriate adjustments to your lifestyle and diet. For example, during the transition from summer to autumn, you may find yourself more susceptible to Vata imbalances. Incorporating Vata-pacifying practices earlier than usual during this transitional period is advisable.

Individual Dosha Considerations:
While these are general guidelines for seasonal adjustments, it's essential to
remember that each individual's constitution and current state of balance are unique. What works for one person may not work for another. Someone with a predominantly Vata constitution will be more sensitive to the Vata-aggravating qualities of autumn, requiring more diligent adherence to Vata-pacifying practices. Similarly, a Pitta-predominant individual will need to pay closer attention to the heat and inflammation potential of the summer months. A Kapha-predominant individual, naturally inclined towards sluggishness, requires additional vigilance during the Kapha-aggravating winter months.

Observing your body's responses is paramount. Pay attention to symptoms such as digestive issues, skin changes, mood swings, energy levels, and sleep patterns. These cues can guide you in making appropriate adjustments to your daily routine, diet, and lifestyle. Keeping a journal to track these changes can be incredibly beneficial.

In conclusion, understanding and adapting to seasonal doshic shifts is a cornerstone of Ayurvedic living. By incorporating these seasonal adjustments into your lifestyle, you can enhance your resilience, promote optimal health, and create a greater harmony between your internal constitution and the ever-changing external world. Remember, Ayurveda is a journey of self-discovery and self-care. Listen to your body, make mindful choices, and enjoy the transformative power of living in sync with the rhythms of nature. This holistic approach will not only enhance your physical health but also foster a deeper connection with your inner self and the natural world around you. The wisdom of Ayurveda lies in its emphasis on preventative care; by proactively adapting to seasonal changes, you are investing in long-term well-being and preventing potential imbalances before they become significant health concerns. This mindful approach allows you to experience the full potential of Ayurveda's holistic healing principles.

Sweet Sour Salty Pungent Bitter Astringent

Ayurveda, the ancient Indian system of medicine, emphasizes the importance of a balanced diet as a cornerstone of health and well-being. Central to this understanding is the concept of the six tastes, or *rasa*, each possessing unique qualities and effects on the body's constitution, or dosha. Understanding and incorporating these six tastes – sweet, sour, salty, pungent, bitter, and astringent – into your daily diet is crucial for maintaining equilibrium and preventing disease. Each taste possesses specific energetic qualities that influence the body's physiological processes, and by consciously balancing these tastes, we can support our individual doshic balance and overall health.

The **sweet taste** (*madhura*), often associated with earth and water elements, is grounding and nourishing. It provides energy, promotes tissue growth, and has a calming effect on the mind. Foods with a sweet taste include grains like rice and barley, most fruits (especially ripe ones), root vegetables such as carrots and sweet potatoes, and dairy products like milk and ghee. However, it's important to distinguish between naturally sweet foods and those loaded with refined sugars. While a small amount of naturally occurring sweetness can be beneficial, excessive consumption of refined sugars can lead to imbalances in the doshas, particularly causing Kapha aggravation and contributing to weight gain and sluggishness. Moderation is key, and choosing whole, unprocessed sweet foods is crucial for reaping the benefits without the drawbacks.

The **sour taste** (*amla*), associated with fire and water, is stimulating and aids digestion. It helps to increase appetite and enhance the function of the digestive fire, or *agni*.

Foods with a sour taste include lemons, limes, tamarinds, yogurt (in moderation, depending on dosha), and certain vinegars. Sour tastes also help increase digestive secretions and promote proper absorption of nutrients, leading to better overall health. However, excessive sour taste can increase Pitta, leading to inflammation and acidity. For those with already aggravated Pitta, limiting the consumption of sour foods can be beneficial. The key is balance and mindful consumption, choosing naturally occurring sour foods in measured quantities.

The **salty taste** (*lavana*), dominated by water, is crucial for maintaining electrolyte balance and hydration. It supports the body's fluid regulation and contributes to proper nerve function. Foods with a salty taste, such as sea salt (in moderation), are essential for various bodily processes, including muscle contraction and nutrient absorption. However, excessive salt consumption can severely aggravate Vata and Pitta, potentially leading to high blood pressure, dehydration, and other health issues. Opting for unprocessed sea salt in minimal quantities is far healthier than relying on processed, refined table salt containing additives and anti-caking agents.

The **pungent taste** (*katu*), characterized by fire and air, is stimulating, cleansing, and excellent for improving digestion. It stimulates the appetite and aids in the removal of toxins, improving the clarity of the mind. Foods with a pungent taste include ginger, garlic, black pepper, chilies, and mustard. Pungent spices are vital for promoting healthy digestion and circulatory function. However, an excessive intake of pungent foods can aggravate Pitta and Vata, potentially causing heat, inflammation, and digestive distress. Balancing the pungent taste by combining it with cooling, sweet, or bitter flavors can mitigate these potential negative effects.

The **bitter taste** (*tikta*), representing space and air, is known for its detoxifying and cooling properties. It helps to cleanse the body, reduce excess heat, and calm the mind.

Foods with a bitter taste include green leafy vegetables, cruciferous vegetables like broccoli and kale, and certain herbs like neem and turmeric. These foods are crucial in supporting healthy liver function and eliminating toxins from the body. While the bitter taste is generally considered good for balancing Pitta, excessive intake can sometimes exacerbate Vata and lead to digestive discomfort. Finding the right balance based on individual constitution is therefore important.

The **astringent taste** (*kashaya*), associated with earth and air, has a drying and constricting effect. It promotes tissue repair, reduces inflammation, and helps to tighten tissues.

Foods with an astringent taste include legumes, beans, pomegranates, cranberries, and certain nuts. These foods can be highly beneficial for controlling diarrhea, bleeding, and reducing excessive secretions. Excessive astringent taste can also cause constipation and aggravate Vata, so balance is crucial.

The skillful combination of these six tastes in a meal is key to Ayurvedic dietary practice. A balanced meal should contain a harmonious blend of all six tastes, although the proportion of each taste will vary depending on the individual's dosha and current state of health. For instance, a Vata-dominant individual might benefit from a diet rich in sweet, sour, and salty tastes, while a Pitta-dominant individual might require more bitter and astringent tastes to counter their fiery nature. A Kapha-dominant individual often benefits from a diet that incorporates more pungent and bitter tastes to stimulate digestion and reduce Kapha accumulation. It's vital to remember that the proportions of each rasa should be balanced to optimize digestion, nutrient absorption, and overall well-being. Furthermore, the seasonal variations should also influence the balance of the six tastes. During hotter months, cooler tastes like bitter and astringent might be favored, while during colder months, warming tastes like sweet and salty may be more beneficial.

The application of the six tastes isn't merely a matter of taste preference; it's a fundamental aspect of balancing the body's energies and maintaining health. By understanding the properties and effects of each taste, and by carefully choosing foods based on both your individual constitution and the season, you can effectively nourish your body and support your overall well-being. A balanced diet, enriched with the wisdom of the six tastes, forms the bedrock of a healthy and harmonious Ayurvedic lifestyle. This conscious approach to eating is not just about sustenance; it's about promoting balance, vitality, and a deeper connection with your body and its intrinsic wisdom. Through mindful selection and thoughtful preparation of food, you can foster a journey towards optimal health and well-being, guided by the time-honored principles of Ayurveda. Remember to consult with a qualified Ayurvedic practitioner for personalized advice, tailored to your unique needs and constitution. They can guide you in creating a diet and lifestyle that aligns perfectly with your dosha and promotes optimal health.

DoshaSpecific Dietary Guidelines

Understanding the unique characteristics of each dosha—Vata, Pitta, and Kapha—is paramount to creating a personalized dietary plan that promotes balance and well-being. While the six tastes offer a foundational framework for Ayurvedic eating, individual dosha needs necessitate a more nuanced approach. Foods that nourish one dosha may aggravate another, highlighting the importance of tailoring your diet to your specific constitution. Let's delve into dosha-specific dietary guidelines, offering insights into food choices that support each dosha's unique energetic profile.

Vata Dosha: Pacifying the Air and Ether

Vata dosha, characterized by air and ether elements, tends towards dryness, lightness, and coolness. Individuals with a predominantly Vata constitution often experience symptoms like constipation, anxiety, insomnia, and dry skin. Their diets should emphasize foods that are warm, moist, grounding, and stable. This means incorporating plenty of cooked foods, avoiding excessive raw foods or salads unless they are combined with warming spices and healthy fats.

Foods to Embrace:
Warm, cooked grains like quinoa, brown rice, and oats provide grounding energy. Soups and stews, especially those featuring root vegetables like carrots, sweet potatoes, and parsnips, offer both warmth and moisture. Legumes such as lentils and chickpeas are excellent sources of protein and fiber, supporting digestive regularity. Healthy fats like ghee (clarified butter), olive oil, and avocado help to lubricate the system and reduce dryness. Sweet fruits like ripe bananas, mangoes, and apples offer soothing energy, while warming spices such as ginger,

cinnamon, and cardamom help to stimulate digestion and circulation. Nuts and seeds, especially sesame seeds and almonds, offer essential fatty acids and minerals. Dairy products, especially warm milk with honey or spices, are also beneficial.

Foods to Limit or Avoid:
Raw vegetables, especially those that are cold or leafy, can increase Vata's dryness. Cold drinks and iced beverages should be minimized. Light, airy foods such as popcorn or very crisp crackers tend to
aggravate Vata. Avoid excessive caffeine and alcohol, which can further disrupt Vata's already delicate equilibrium. Spicy and pungent foods in excess can also upset the balance. Skip highly processed foods, refined sugars, and excessive amounts of dried fruits, which lack moisture.

Pitta Dosha: Cooling the Fire

Pitta, characterized by the elements of fire and water, is associated with metabolism, digestion, and transformation. Individuals with a Pitta constitution often possess a fiery temperament, are prone to anger or frustration, and may experience heartburn, ulcers, or skin inflammation. Their diets require a cooling and soothing approach, focusing on foods that reduce heat and inflammation.

Foods to Embrace:
Cooling fruits like watermelon,
cucumber, and coconut offer refreshing hydration. Leafy green vegetables, such as spinach and kale (in moderation), provide essential nutrients without excessive heat. Sweet fruits, such as apples and pears, also offer a gentle sweetness without exacerbating Pitta. Mung beans are easily digestible and cooling. Avoid over-spiced dishes and opt for gentle spices like coriander and fennel. Ghee, in moderation, can also be beneficial, but avoid over-consumption. Sweet potatoes are a good source of energy.

Foods to Limit or Avoid:
Highly acidic foods such as tomatoes, citrus fruits (in large quantities), and vinegar can exacerbate Pitta imbalances. Hot, spicy foods, including chili peppers, garlic (in large quantities), and onions (in large quantities) should be consumed sparingly, or avoided entirely. Avoid overly fermented foods, as they may stimulate digestive fire too intensely. Reduce intake of alcohol and caffeine, as they are known stimulants for Pitta.

Kapha Dosha: Stimulating the Earth and Water

Kapha, characterized by the elements of earth and water, is associated with stability, structure, and lubrication. Individuals with a Kapha constitution are often grounded, stable, and resilient, but may struggle with weight gain, sluggishness, or respiratory congestion. Their diets should emphasize lighter, warming, and stimulating foods that help to enhance metabolism and promote lightness.

Foods to Embrace:
Light and easily digestible foods like barley and millet are preferable to heavier grains such as rice. Spices such as ginger, cinnamon, and black pepper stimulate digestion and help to reduce Kapha's tendency towards stagnation. Bitter vegetables like broccoli and asparagus promote healthy elimination. Pungent spices such as mustard seeds or radish are good for Kapha types. Light vegetables like zucchini, turnips, and radishes are better options compared to heavy starchy vegetables. Consume fruits in moderation and avoid sweet, heavy fruits like bananas and mangoes.

Foods to Limit or Avoid:
Avoid heavy, rich, and oily foods as they can further increase Kapha's inherent heaviness. Dairy products should be consumed in moderation. Reduce intake of sweet and oily foods as these can increase Kapha

buildup. Avoid excessive amounts of fatty meats and deep-fried foods. Minimize intake of refined sugars, as they lead to energy imbalances and weigh down the system. Limit consumption of heavy, dense grains such as rice and wheat, opting for lighter alternatives. Reduce consumption of root vegetables, as these can be heavy and dampening for Kapha.

Seasonal Adjustments

It's crucial to remember that these are general guidelines, and seasonal considerations play a critical role in maintaining doshic balance. During colder months, it's generally advisable to incorporate more warming and grounding foods, while in warmer months, cooler and lighter foods are often preferred. Consulting an Ayurvedic practitioner can provide personalized recommendations based on your specific dosha, current state of health, and the prevailing season.

For example, a Vata individual might increase their intake of warming spices and root vegetables during winter, while a Pitta individual might prioritize cooling fruits and vegetables during summer. A Kapha person may need to consume lighter, more stimulating foods throughout the year but especially during the wetter, cooler months when Kapha tends to be more dominant.

Beyond Food:

Dietary considerations form a vital part of Ayurvedic wellness but it is only one element. The six tastes act as a guiding principle, informing food choices, but a holistic approach also incorporates lifestyle factors such as exercise (yoga, pranayama), sleep patterns, stress management techniques (meditation, mindfulness), and daily routines (dinacharya). By integrating these practices, you create a comprehensive approach to well-being, ensuring that the positive effects of your tailored diet are amplified and sustained.

Remember that personalized guidance from a qualified Ayurvedic practitioner is invaluable in determining your unique dosha and creating a dietary and lifestyle plan that perfectly aligns with your individual constitution. They can help you navigate the complexities of Ayurvedic nutrition and integrate it seamlessly into your life, promoting a journey of vibrant health and well-being. Don't hesitate to seek professional guidance to harness the full potential of Ayurvedic principles for a healthier, more balanced life. The journey towards optimal health and wellness is a personalized one, requiring careful attention to your unique needs and constitution, and consistent dedication to a balanced lifestyle.

Practical Tips and Examples

Building upon the understanding of doshas and their unique dietary needs, let's explore practical strategies for creating balanced meals that incorporate the six tastes. Remember, the goal isn't rigid adherence to rules, but rather a mindful approach to nourishing your body in a way that promotes balance and vitality. The six tastes – sweet, sour, salty, pungent, bitter, and astringent – each possess unique qualities and effects on the body. A balanced meal incorporates all six tastes, though the proportions will vary depending on your predominant dosha and seasonal influences. Consuming all six tastes in each meal is not always practical or even desirable, but aiming for a balanced distribution throughout the day is key.

For Vata dosha, which is characterized by dryness, coldness, and lightness, the focus should be on warming, grounding, and moistening foods. Sweet, sour, and salty tastes are particularly beneficial for balancing Vata. Think warm, cooked grains like quinoa or brown rice, root vegetables like sweet potatoes and carrots, and warming spices like ginger and cinnamon. Incorporating healthy fats like ghee or coconut oil adds moisture and grounding qualities. Soups and stews are excellent choices for Vata, providing warmth and moisture. A sample Vata-balancing meal could include a warm lentil soup with quinoa, roasted sweet potatoes, and a sprinkle of cinnamon.

Pitta dosha, known for its fiery nature, thrives on cooling and soothing foods. Sweet, bitter, and astringent tastes are particularly beneficial for balancing Pitta. Cooling fruits like watermelon and cucumber, leafy green vegetables, and calming herbs like coriander and mint are ideal choices.

Avoid excessive spices and overly hot foods, which can exacerbate Pitta's fiery nature. A balanced Pitta meal might consist of a salad with cucumber, mint, and coriander, quinoa or brown rice, and a side of steamed green beans. Opt for lighter cooking methods like steaming or grilling to avoid further increasing Pitta's heat. Coconut water is an excellent choice of beverage for Pitta.

Kapha dosha, characterized by heaviness, coolness, and stability, benefits from lighter, warming, and pungent foods. Pungent, bitter, and astringent tastes help to balance Kapha's tendency toward stagnation. Light, easily digestible foods are crucial. Think lighter grains like barley or millet, vegetables like broccoli and asparagus, and warming spices like black pepper or ginger. A balanced Kapha meal could feature a barley porridge with sauteed broccoli, asparagus, and a touch of black pepper. Focus on reducing the consumption of heavier foods, dairy products, and excessively sweet foods that can aggravate Kapha. A light vegetable broth or green tea are ideal beverage choices.

Creating balanced meals extends beyond simply incorporating the six tastes. The cooking methods employed also play a significant role. Steaming, baking, and boiling are generally preferable to frying, which can add excessive heat and create an imbalance in the doshas. The principle of digestion (Agni) is central to Ayurvedic nutrition. If Agni is weak, digestion is compromised, leading to an accumulation of ama (toxins). To support strong Agni, combine foods wisely. Heavy foods should be digested separately from light foods. For instance, do not combine dairy products with starchy vegetables. It's important to incorporate easily digestible and lighter foods into the meal when heavy foods are consumed.

Consider the seasonal influence when planning your meals. In the cooler months, emphasize warming foods, such as soups and stews, whereas in the warmer months, opt for lighter, cooling dishes, such as salads and smoothies. Seasonal fruits and vegetables are naturally the most appropriate and beneficial for the body. This aligns with the principles of nature and its impact on our health.

Let's illustrate this further with specific meal examples, tailored to each dosha:

Vata-Balancing Meal Plan (Autumn/Winter):

Breakfast:
Warm oatmeal with raisins, a sprinkle of cinnamon, and a dollop of ghee. A cup of warm milk with a pinch of cardamom.
Lunch:
Lentil soup with sweet potatoes, carrots, and ginger. A side of quinoa.
Dinner:
Baked sweet potatoes stuffed with black beans, brown rice, and a small amount of cheese.

Pitta-Balancing Meal Plan (Summer):

Breakfast:
Smoothie made with coconut water, cucumber, mint, and a little bit of honey.
Lunch:
Salad with leafy greens, cucumber, sprouts, and a light lemon dressing. A small portion of brown rice.
Dinner:
Steamed green beans, zucchini, and a side of barley.

Kapha-Balancing Meal Plan (Spring):

Breakfast:
Porridge of millet with a pinch of black pepper and a few berries.

Lunch:
Salad with broccoli, asparagus, and a light vinaigrette. A small portion of barley.

Dinner:
Baked vegetables like broccoli, carrots, and cauliflower with a light drizzle of olive oil.

Remember, these are just examples; the best approach is to experiment and find what works best for you. Pay attention to how different foods make you feel. If you experience heaviness, bloating, or other digestive discomfort, you might need to adjust your diet. Keeping a food journal can be incredibly helpful in tracking your food intake, noticing patterns, and identifying foods that may be causing issues.

Beyond the individual dosha considerations, there are several general principles to keep in mind when creating balanced meals:

Mindful Eating:
Eat slowly, savoring each bite. Avoid distractions like television or computers. This promotes better digestion and allows your body to properly process the nutrients from your food.

Variety:
Incorporate a wide range of fruits, vegetables, grains, and legumes into your diet. This ensures a diverse intake of nutrients.

Fresh Foods:
Fresh, seasonal produce is always the best option. It retains its natural nutrients and vitality.

Proper Cooking:
Opt for gentler cooking methods like steaming, baking, and boiling to preserve the nutrients and avoid excessive heat.

Water Intake:
Drink plenty of water throughout the day to support hydration and digestion.

Portion Control:
Pay attention to your portion sizes. Eat until you are comfortably satisfied, not overly full.

The creation of balanced meals is a dynamic process. It requires awareness, observation, and a willingness to adapt and adjust based on your individual needs and how your body responds. Remember to consult with a qualified

Ayurvedic practitioner for personalized guidance, especially if you have any underlying health conditions. They can provide tailored advice based on your unique constitution and health goals, leading you towards a path of vibrant wellness. The journey to Ayurvedic balance is not a destination, but a continual process of mindful nourishment and self-discovery. By understanding the six tastes and their effect on your dosha, you can create meals that support your body's natural rhythms and promote overall well-being.

Delicious and Nourishing Meals

Let's embark on a culinary journey, exploring delicious and nourishing meals tailored to each dosha. Remember, these recipes are guidelines; feel free to adjust spices and ingredients to suit your palate and preferences. The key is to incorporate the six tastes in a balanced way that resonates with your body. Always prioritize fresh, seasonal ingredients whenever possible, for optimal taste and nutritional value.

Vata-Pacifying Recipes:

Vata dosha is characterized by its airy and dry nature, making it susceptible to dryness, anxiety, and digestive issues. Vata-pacifying meals should be warm, moist, grounding, and rich in healthy fats.

Warm Quinoa Salad with Roasted Vegetables and Toasted Nuts:

This recipe combines the grounding qualities of quinoa with the sweetness of roasted root vegetables and the healthy fats from nuts and seeds. Roast butternut squash, sweet potatoes, and carrots until tender. Toss with cooked quinoa, toasted walnuts and pumpkin seeds, and a dressing of olive oil, maple syrup, and a pinch of cinnamon. This dish incorporates sweet, salty, and slightly bitter tastes, creating a comforting and balancing meal. The warmth of the roasted vegetables further soothes Vata.

Lentil Soup with Coconut Milk:

Lentils are a wonderful source of protein and fiber, perfect for stabilizing Vata. This hearty soup combines red lentils, coconut milk, warming spices like ginger and turmeric, and a touch of sea salt. The coconut milk adds richness and moisture, counteracting Vata's dryness. Consider adding a dollop of ghee (clarified butter) for an extra layer of richness and warmth. The combination of sweet, salty, and pungent tastes promotes digestion and provides grounding nourishment.

Oatmeal with Apples and Cinnamon:
A warm bowl of oatmeal is incredibly soothing for Vata. Cook oatmeal with water or milk, and add diced apples, a sprinkle of cinnamon, and a drizzle of honey or maple syrup. The sweetness, warmth, and grounding nature of this breakfast bowl help calm the nervous system and provide sustained energy throughout the morning. The added fiber promotes healthy digestion.

Pitta-Balancing Recipes:

Pitta, characterized by fire and water elements, benefits from cooling, calming, and slightly sweet meals. Avoid overly spicy or acidic foods.

Cucumber and Mint Raita:
This cooling and refreshing raita is perfect for balancing Pitta's fiery nature. Combine grated cucumber, fresh mint, a squeeze of lime juice (use sparingly), and a dollop of plain yogurt. This dish provides a delightful combination of sweet, sour, and astringent tastes, offering a soothing and digestive aid. The coolness of the cucumber and mint helps to calm Pitta's intensity.

Basmati Rice with Steamed Green Vegetables:
Basmati rice is a lighter grain compared to other rice varieties, better suited to Pitta's constitution. Serve it with steamed green vegetables like broccoli, asparagus, or green beans. This meal offers a balanced combination of the six tastes, with the emphasis on the sweet, slightly bitter, and astringent tastes to balance Pitta's heat.

Coconut Milk and Mango Smoothie:
A creamy and
naturally sweet smoothie is an excellent way to nourish a Pitta dosha. Combine coconut milk, ripe mango, a touch of lime juice (use cautiously), and a pinch of cardamom. This smoothie is both cooling and hydrating, offering a delightful balance of sweet, sour, and slightly pungent tastes. The coolness of the coconut milk and mango helps reduce Pitta's fiery energy.

Kapha-Reducing Recipes:

Kapha, characterized by earth and water, thrives on lighter, warming, and slightly pungent meals to stimulate digestion and reduce stagnation.

Spiced Chickpea Salad:
This light and flavorful salad combines chickpeas, chopped vegetables (such as bell
peppers, onions, and cucumbers), and a dressing of lemon juice, olive oil, and a blend of warming spices like cumin, coriander, and turmeric. The pungent and bitter notes from the spices stimulate digestion and promote a sense of lightness. The balance of tastes ensures proper nourishment.

Ginger-Garlic Greens:
Sautéed leafy green vegetables (like spinach, kale, or mustard greens) with fresh ginger and garlic are a light and warming option for Kapha. The pungent taste from ginger and garlic aids digestion, and the bitter taste from the greens helps balance the heavy nature of Kapha. A sprinkle of red pepper flakes can further stimulate the
digestive fire.

Mung Bean Soup with Lemon:
Mung beans are easily digestible and considered a light protein source for Kapha. This soup is best made with minimal oil and seasoned with lemon juice for a sour and slightly astringent kick to promote

digestion. Include spices such as cumin and coriander to improve digestion further.

Seasonal Considerations:

Remember to adapt your meals to the changing seasons. In the warmer months, opt for lighter, cooling dishes, while during colder months, embrace warm, grounding recipes. For example, during summer, focus on cooling fruits like watermelon and cucumber, while during winter, consider adding warming spices like ginger and cinnamon to your meals.

Recipe Variations and Customization:

These are just starting points; feel free to adapt these recipes to your taste and dietary needs. Experiment with different spices, herbs, and vegetables to find what works best for your body. You can also substitute ingredients based on availability and personal preference. The goal is to find a balance of tastes that nourishes and satisfies you.

Importance of mindful eating:

Beyond the recipes themselves, remember the importance of mindful eating. Eat slowly, savoring each bite, and paying attention to your body's signals of hunger and fullness. This mindful approach to eating enhances digestion and promotes overall well-being, complementing the benefits of balanced Ayurvedic meals. Creating a calm and peaceful environment during mealtimes further enhances the digestive process and allows for better assimilation of nutrients.

Beyond the Plate:

Ayurvedic nutrition isn't solely about the food we eat; it's about the entire experience of eating. Consider the following:

Preparation:
The way you prepare your food impacts its energetic qualities. Use fresh, organic ingredients whenever possible, and approach cooking with intention and care.

Presentation:
The way you present your food can also enhance your dining experience. Use attractive serving dishes and take your time creating visually appealing meals.

Company:
Sharing meals with loved ones can be a powerful way to enhance digestion and nurture your social well-being.

By integrating these principles into your daily life, you can move beyond simply consuming food to truly nourishing your body and spirit through the holistic wisdom of Ayurveda. The journey towards balanced eating is a continuous process of exploration, adjustment, and mindful appreciation of the food that fuels your body and supports your unique constitution. Remember to listen to your body, adjust your meals as needed, and consult a qualified Ayurvedic practitioner for personalized guidance. This journey towards holistic well-being is a personal one, and with conscious effort and mindful practice, you can achieve a vibrant and healthy life through the principles of Ayurvedic nutrition.

Adapting Your Diet to the Changing Seasons

Ayurveda emphasizes the profound connection between our internal balance and the rhythms of nature. Just as the seasons shift and change, so too should our dietary choices to maintain harmony within our bodies. Seasonal eating, a cornerstone of Ayurvedic nutrition, is about aligning our food intake with the prevailing energies of each season. This approach not only enhances the nutritional value of our meals but also promotes a deeper connection to the natural world, fostering a sense of well-being that extends beyond the purely physical.

Spring, the season of renewal, is characterized by the burgeoning of life. The air becomes lighter, warmer, and filled with the sweet fragrance of blooming flowers. Our bodies, too, respond to this energetic shift. During spring, Vata dosha tends to be more prominent, needing grounding. Therefore, it's advisable to focus on warm, cooked foods that are moist and nourishing. Think hearty soups featuring root vegetables like carrots, parsnips, and sweet potatoes. Spices such as ginger and turmeric can further aid digestion and combat any lingering Vata imbalances from the colder months. Light, leafy greens like spinach and kale, rich in vitamins and minerals, are also ideal. Avoid excessive consumption of raw salads, which can further increase Vata. Incorporate warming oils like ghee or coconut oil into your cooking to enhance the digestive process and provide essential fatty acids. This approach helps to counter the dryness often associated with Vata dosha during this transitional season.

Summer, with its intense heat, brings its own set of dietary considerations. Pitta dosha, characterized by fire and transformation, tends to become aggravated during this season. Therefore, cooling and pacifying foods are essential. Light, easily digestible meals are key. Salads featuring cucumber, mint, and coriander are excellent choices, offering a refreshing contrast to the summer's heat. Fruits like watermelon, berries, and mangoes are not only delicious but also provide vital hydration. Avoid hot and spicy foods that could further inflame Pitta. Opt for foods that are sweet, bitter, and astringent in taste to balance the fiery nature of summer. Remember to stay well-hydrated by drinking plenty of water, infused with cooling herbs like basil or mint. This approach helps to prevent overheating and maintain internal equilibrium during the hottest months of the year. Consider incorporating cooling herbs such as fennel and cilantro into your daily meals to help soothe Pitta. Also, try reducing the consumption of alcohol and caffeine during the summer to avoid further aggravating the dosha. Choosing lighter meals, such as soups or stews made with lighter vegetables, can also ease the digestive burden, which is often compromised in the summer.

Autumn, with its crisp air and changing colors, marks a period of transition. As the days grow shorter and the temperature drops, Kapha dosha may become more prominent. The emphasis in autumn is on balancing the increased heaviness associated with Kapha. This is the time to incorporate lighter, easily digestible foods. Include more warming spices such as cinnamon, cloves, and cardamom to stimulate digestion and metabolic function. Embrace root vegetables like butternut squash and sweet potatoes, which provide warmth and essential nutrients. Beans, lentils, and rice are also excellent options, providing complex carbohydrates that sustain energy levels during the cooler months. Aim for a balance of light and grounding foods, avoiding excessive intake of foods that are heavy, oily, or overly sweet. This careful balance ensures that your system maintains its equilibrium as it prepares for the winter ahead. Consider using warming herbs and spices in your tea and cooking. The warmth and flavor boost your energy levels and aid digestion. This transitional time calls for a balanced diet that prepares the body for the coming cold weather.

Winter, characterized by its cold and often dry climate, demands a dietary approach that provides warmth, nourishment, and protection. The emphasis is on foods that are rich, warm, and comforting. Stews, soups, and warm porridges made with nourishing grains like barley and oats are especially suitable. Incorporate warming spices such as ginger, cinnamon, cloves, and black pepper to enhance digestion and stimulate circulation. Root vegetables, such as carrots, beets, and turnips, are excellent sources of essential nutrients during these colder months. Incorporating healthy fats from sources like ghee and nuts also helps to maintain warmth and protect against the cold. Avoid excessively cold foods and drinks, as they can further cool the body and aggravate Vata. By embracing these principles, you ensure your body receives the support it needs to stay healthy and resilient throughout the cold season. Consider adding warming oils, such as sesame or mustard, to your cooking to enhance the warmth of your meals. These choices will be particularly beneficial during the colder months and aid in maintaining optimal bodily warmth and function. A warming beverage before bed, such as warm milk with turmeric and ginger, will further enhance warmth and relaxation.

Beyond these seasonal guidelines, Ayurveda emphasizes the importance of mindful eating. Paying attention to your body's signals of hunger and satiety, chewing your food thoroughly, and eating in a relaxed atmosphere are all crucial aspects of optimal digestion and nourishment. Avoid eating while distracted, such as while working or watching television. Remember that seasonal eating is not merely about consuming specific foods but about embracing the philosophy of aligning your diet with the natural rhythms of the environment. By adapting your diet to the seasonal changes, you foster a harmonious relationship between your body and nature, enhancing your overall health and well-being. This conscious engagement with your diet transforms the act of eating from a simple necessity into a mindful and nourishing experience, creating a deeper connection between you and your food. The subtle shifts in taste and texture, the seasonal abundance, and the simple pleasure of savoring the flavors of the moment will contribute to a greater appreciation for the food that sustains you.

Furthermore, consider the impact of local and seasonal produce on your health. Locally sourced ingredients are fresher, contain more nutrients, and generally have a lower environmental impact. By choosing seasonal fruits and vegetables, you're not only aligning your diet with the natural rhythms of the earth but also supporting sustainable agriculture. This mindful approach to food procurement is a vital aspect of a holistic Ayurvedic lifestyle.

The importance of adapting your spice and herb choices according to the season cannot be overstated. Ayurvedic cooking heavily emphasizes spices and herbs not just for flavor but for their medicinal properties. During the cooler months, warming spices like ginger, cinnamon, and cloves aid digestion and improve circulation. In warmer months, cooling spices such as coriander, mint, and fennel counteract the heat. This careful selection of spices and herbs further supports the seasonal adaptation of your diet. Experiment with different spice combinations and find those that resonate most with your body and palate. The subtle changes in flavors and the therapeutic benefits they offer will further enhance your culinary journey.

The principle of seasonal eating extends beyond simply incorporating specific foods; it also involves understanding the energy and qualities of each season. Spring's energy is characterized by lightness and growth, prompting a focus on lighter and less-dense foods. Autumn's energy shifts towards grounding and preparation for winter, leading to a focus on denser and more grounding foods. Summer's heat calls for cooling foods, while winter's cold requires warming and nourishing foods. This understanding allows for a deeper and more intuitive approach to dietary choices. Observe how your body responds to different foods throughout the year. This intimate understanding of your body's responses to seasonal changes will further refine your seasonal eating practice.

Finally, seasonal eating is a journey, not a destination. It's about continuous observation, experimentation, and mindful adaptation. As you become more attuned to the rhythms of nature and the needs of your body, your seasonal diet will evolve, becoming a personalized reflection of your unique constitution and the season at hand. Consult with a qualified Ayurvedic practitioner for personalized guidance on adapting your diet to suit your specific dosha and the prevailing seasonal energies. This guidance will further optimize your dietary choices and ensure that they are perfectly aligned with your individual needs and the demands of the seasons. Remember that the principles of Ayurveda emphasize balance and harmony, both within your body and with the natural world. Through mindful adaptation, seasonal eating becomes a potent tool for promoting wellness and a profound connection with the Earth.

Setting the Tone for a Balanced Day

The day begins long before the sun crests the horizon. In Ayurveda, the dawn is not just a marker of time, but a potent opportunity to set the tone for the entire day. The ancient practice of *Dinacharya*, the daily routine, emphasizes this, and its morning rituals are particularly crucial in establishing a foundation of balance and well-being. Neglecting these seemingly small practices can subtly undermine our health, leaving us vulnerable to imbalances over time. Conversely, diligently following them can create a ripple effect of positive energy, impacting not just our physical health, but our mental clarity, emotional stability, and overall sense of well-being.

The first step in this transformative process is to awaken gently, ideally before sunrise. This allows us to connect with the natural rhythm of the day, harmonizing ourselves with the earth's energy. Rushing into the day without this mindful transition can instantly create a state of internal chaos, setting the stage for stress and imbalance. Instead, try to awaken naturally, without the jarring sound of an alarm clock if possible. If an alarm is necessary, opt for a gentle chime or natural sounds rather than a harsh, abrupt tone. Take a few moments to simply lie in bed, observing your breath, and gently stretching your limbs. This conscious transition from sleep to wakefulness cultivates a sense of calm and prepares the body and mind for the day ahead.

Next, we move to the practice of *Jala Neti*, or nasal cleansing. This simple yet profoundly effective technique uses a neti pot—a small teapot-like vessel—to gently irrigate the nasal passages with warm, salted water. It removes accumulated mucus, dust, and other impurities, effectively clearing the nasal passages and improving breathing. This is particularly important for those prone to allergies or respiratory issues, but its benefits extend far beyond symptom relief. By clearing the nasal pathways, we improve the quality of our prana, or life force energy, allowing for clearer thinking and enhanced sensory perception. Furthermore, it's a gentle form of detoxification, removing toxins that might otherwise accumulate and affect our overall health. The act of Jala Neti itself is a meditative practice, fostering a sense of mindfulness and cleansing even beyond the physical level.

Following nasal cleansing, we turn to *Jihwa Prakarshanam*, or tongue scraping. This involves using a specially designed tongue scraper to gently remove the white coating that often accumulates on the tongue overnight. This coating, called *ama* in Ayurveda, is composed of accumulated toxins and bacteria. Removing it not only improves oral hygiene and freshens breath, but also aids in removing toxins from the body, improving digestion, and even potentially reducing the risk of certain diseases. The process is remarkably straightforward and takes mere seconds. It involves gently scraping the tongue from back to front, rinsing the scraper thoroughly after each swipe, and ultimately rinsing your mouth with warm water. The simple act of tongue scraping can dramatically improve your sense of taste and overall oral health.

The next ritual, *Gandusha*, or oil pulling, is a technique that has gained widespread popularity in recent years. This ancient Ayurvedic practice involves swishing a tablespoon of oil, typically sesame or coconut oil, in the mouth for 15-20 minutes before rinsing and spitting it out. The oil acts as a natural detoxifier, drawing out impurities and bacteria from the mouth and gums. While the scientific community is still exploring the full range of its benefits, many proponents report improvements in oral health, including whiter teeth, reduced gum inflammation, and improved overall oral hygiene. Furthermore, some individuals report feeling a boost in energy and a clearer mind after the practice. While there's some debate about the extent of its systemic effects, its impact on oral health alone makes it a worthwhile addition to any morning routine.

Next is
Abhyanga
, the practice of self-massage with warm, medicated oil. This is not just a luxurious indulgence, but a powerful therapeutic practice that nourishes the skin,
balances the doshas, and promotes relaxation. The warm oil lubricates the joints, improves circulation, and soothes the nervous system. The massage itself can be adapted to suit individual needs and preferences. Some individuals prefer a gentle, soothing massage, while others opt for a more vigorous approach. Regardless of the intensity, the act of self-massage is a powerful way to connect with the body, to appreciate its physicality and to honor its needs. The specific oil used should ideally be chosen based on individual dosha. For instance, sesame oil is often recommended for Vata dosha, while coconut oil may suit Pitta dosha. The warmth of the oil and the act of massage itself contribute to relaxation and can be a significant aid in reducing stress levels and promoting better sleep.

After Abhyanga, it is recommended to take a warm shower or bath. This removes the excess oil used in the massage and leaves the skin feeling clean and refreshed. This is also a time for mindful reflection, offering a transition between the more introspective practices of the early morning and the more outward-focused demands of the day.

Finally, before beginning the day's activities, it is vital to consume a warm beverage. This could be a cup of herbal tea (like ginger or turmeric tea), a small bowl of warm water, or even just a glass of room temperature water with lemon. This helps to rehydrate the body and awaken the digestive system, preparing it for the day's nourishment. Avoiding cold drinks or foods first thing in the morning is important, as these can dampen the digestive fire and leave one feeling sluggish and lethargic.

These morning rituals, although seemingly simple, represent a profound shift in our relationship with ourselves and the natural world. They are not merely steps in a routine, but rather intentional acts of self-care, each designed to cultivate balance, energy, and vitality. By incorporating these practices into our daily lives, we lay the groundwork for a day filled with clarity, focus, and well-being, setting the stage for a life lived in harmony with nature's rhythms and our own unique constitution. It's crucial to remember that the key to success with Dinacharya is consistency and personalization. Start with one or two practices that resonate with you, and gradually incorporate others as you feel comfortable. Over time, these rituals will become an integral part of your daily life, and the benefits will be truly transformative. The key is not to view these practices as burdensome tasks, but as acts of self-love and devotion, a sacred offering to the temple of your own body and mind. The rewards—enhanced physical and mental well-being, increased energy, and a profound sense of inner peace—are worth the time and effort invested in establishing this powerful foundation for a healthy and fulfilling life.

Maintaining Energy and Focus

The midday sun bears down, and the energy that propelled you through the morning may begin to wane. This is a natural rhythm, a dip in the energetic arc of the day, and understanding this is key to navigating the afternoon with grace and maintaining focus and productivity. Ayurveda offers a range of practices designed to counteract this natural afternoon slump, ensuring you can maintain equilibrium and vitality until the day's close. These practices are not about forcing energy where there is none, but rather about working *with*
the body's natural ebb and flow, supporting its inherent capacity for self-regulation.

One of the most crucial afternoon practices is rest. This doesn't necessarily mean a full-blown nap, although a short, 20-minute restorative rest can be incredibly beneficial, especially for Vata types prone to exhaustion. For others, a simple period of quiet contemplation can be equally effective. This could involve sitting comfortably, closing your eyes, and focusing on your breath. Even five to ten minutes of quietude can make a significant difference in restoring mental clarity and reducing fatigue. The aim is to allow the body and mind to gently downshift, a necessary counterpoint to the demands of the day. This is not laziness; it's an act of self-preservation, a strategic retreat to recharge and replenish before tackling the remaining tasks.

The type of rest you choose should align with your doshic constitution. Vata types, characterized by their airy and mobile nature, often benefit from gentle, grounding activities during the afternoon. A short meditation, a warm bath infused with calming essential oils like lavender or chamomile, or even a few minutes spent listening to soothing music can help anchor their restless energy. Pitta individuals, with their fiery and passionate nature, often benefit from cooling activities. A cool shower, a light walk in the shade, or consuming a cooling beverage like coconut water can help temper their inner heat and prevent burnout. Kapha types, characterized by their earthy and grounded nature, may benefit from gentle movement to stimulate their energy levels. A short walk or some light stretching can help counteract the tendency towards sluggishness that can arise in the afternoon.

Mindful movement is another powerful tool for maintaining afternoon energy and focus. This doesn't require a strenuous workout; gentle exercise is often more beneficial at this time of day. A brisk walk in nature, a short session of yoga, or even some simple stretches at your desk can help improve circulation, boost energy levels, and alleviate mental fatigue. The focus here is on gentle movement that encourages relaxation and rejuvenation, not intense exertion that can deplete energy further. Choose activities that are calming and restorative, such as Tai Chi or Qi Gong, which combine gentle movement with mindful breathing and meditation. These practices can help to center your mind, release tension, and promote a sense of calm and well-being. Even a few sun salutations (Surya Namaskar) can revitalize your energy levels and enhance your focus.

Proper hydration is paramount throughout the day, but it's especially important in the afternoon to combat dehydration, a common cause of fatigue and reduced cognitive function. Water is the best choice, but you can also incorporate herbal teas that support your dosha. For example, cooling teas like rose or jasmine can be beneficial for Pitta individuals, while warming teas like ginger or chamomile can be helpful for Vata and Kapha types. Avoid excessive caffeine or sugary drinks in the afternoon, as these can lead to an energy crash later on. Opt for naturally hydrating options, such as coconut water, watermelon juice, or cucumber slices infused in water for a refreshing and revitalizing treat. The timing of your hydration is crucial too. Sipping water throughout the afternoon is far more beneficial than gulping down a large quantity at once. Allowing the body to gradually absorb the water will maintain optimal hydration levels without the potential sluggishness that may result from large quantities consumed immediately.

Dietary choices significantly impact your afternoon energy levels. Avoid heavy, greasy meals, which can lead to sluggishness and digestive discomfort. Opt for lighter, easily digestible foods, such as soups, salads, or vegetable stir-fries. Include a variety of fresh fruits and vegetables to provide essential nutrients and support healthy digestion. A balanced meal with a focus on whole grains, lean proteins, and plenty of vegetables is an excellent choice to maintain your energy levels throughout the afternoon. Remember the six tastes of Ayurveda: sweet, sour, salty, pungent, bitter, and astringent. Aim for a balanced combination of tastes to support healthy digestion and prevent imbalances. A small, mindful snack in the late afternoon can stave off cravings and prevent a sudden energy drop. Choose a snack that is easy to digest and nourishing, such as a handful of nuts, a piece of fruit, or a small bowl of yogurt. Avoid processed snacks, as they often lead to an energy crash.

Maintaining optimal energy levels in the afternoon also involves creating a supportive environment. Ensure you have adequate lighting, good ventilation, and a clutter-free workspace. These small changes to your surroundings can have a significant impact on your ability to focus and maintain productivity. A change of scenery can also be effective. If possible, step outside for a few minutes to get some fresh air and sunlight. This can help to boost your mood and energy levels. Even a brief walk around the block can make a difference.

Beyond the physical practices, the mental and emotional aspects of your afternoon routine are equally important. Practicing mindfulness throughout the day, even in small moments, can help to prevent mental fatigue and maintain focus. Take a few moments to pause and appreciate the present moment, noticing your breath, your surroundings, and your feelings without judgment. Simple acts of self-care, such as taking a few deep breaths, listening to calming music, or stretching your body, can significantly contribute to your overall well-being. This mental and emotional attention is integral to managing energy through the day, as the mind and body are intrinsically connected within the Ayurvedic framework.

Integrating Ayurvedic principles into your afternoon routine doesn't require a complete overhaul of your lifestyle. Start by incorporating one or two practices that resonate with you and gradually add others as you become comfortable. The key is consistency. Making these practices a regular part of your routine will help you maintain energy, focus, and overall well-being throughout the afternoon. Remember that the afternoon dip is natural; it's how you respond to it that shapes the rest of your day. By embracing the principles of Ayurveda, you equip yourself with the tools to not only survive this natural lull, but to thrive through the remainder of the day feeling balanced, focused and energized. The beauty of Ayurveda lies in its adaptability; find what works best for your unique constitution and make it your own. Over time, these seemingly simple practices will accumulate, shaping a life characterized by vitality, clarity, and a deep sense of inner harmony.

Preparing for Restful Sleep

As the sun dips below the horizon, painting the sky in hues of orange and purple, it's time to transition from the day's activities into a state of calm and preparation for restful sleep. The evening routine, or *Sandhya Dinacharya*, is a crucial element of Ayurvedic daily practice, designed to gently unwind the body and mind, promoting a deep and restorative sleep. This is not merely about falling asleep; it's about cultivating a peaceful transition into the regenerative phase of the circadian rhythm. The quality of your sleep profoundly impacts your overall health and well-being, influencing everything from digestion and immunity to mood and cognitive function. A well-structured evening routine, tailored to your individual doshic constitution, can significantly enhance the quality of your sleep and, consequently, your overall health.

The first step in preparing for sleep is to begin winding down at least an hour or two before your intended bedtime. This transition period is crucial to allow your body to naturally reduce its activity levels and prepare for rest. Avoid engaging in strenuous activities or stimulating mental tasks during this time. Instead, opt for calming activities that promote relaxation and tranquility. The light emitted from electronic devices, such as smartphones, tablets, and computers, significantly impacts melatonin production, a hormone crucial for regulating sleep. Therefore, minimizing screen time in the hour or two before bed is highly recommended. Consider replacing this screen time with activities that promote relaxation, such as reading a physical book, listening to calming music, or gentle stretching.

For Vata individuals, characterized by their airy and ethereal nature, the evening routine requires extra care to establish a sense of grounding and stability. Their tendency towards anxiety and restlessness necessitates a gentle approach to relaxation. A warm bath infused with essential oils such as lavender or chamomile can be incredibly soothing. The warm water helps to relax tense muscles, while the calming aroma of the essential oils further promotes relaxation and reduces anxiety. A gentle massage with warm sesame oil can also be highly beneficial. This practice, known as *Abhyanga*, helps to lubricate the joints and calm the nervous system, preparing the body for sleep. Vatas should also prioritize creating a warm and cozy sleep environment, avoiding cold temperatures and drafts. A regular bedtime routine, devoid of rushed activity, is crucial, along with avoiding late-night meals and caffeinated beverages.

Pitta individuals, known for their fiery and passionate nature, often experience difficulty unwinding due to their naturally high energy levels. Their evening routine should emphasize cooling and calming practices. A cool shower or bath can help to reduce body temperature and calm the mind. The avoidance of stimulating foods and activities is also important. Spicy foods, intense exercise, and stressful conversations should be minimized in the hours leading up to bedtime. Instead, focus on calming activities like light yoga, meditation, or listening to soothing music. Pitta types benefit greatly from practices that encourage a sense of mental quietude. Journaling can be a helpful outlet for processing thoughts and emotions, preventing racing thoughts from disturbing sleep. The consistent practice of Pranayama (yogic breathing techniques), particularly calming techniques like Ujjayi breath, can significantly contribute to reducing Pitta's fiery intensity and promoting relaxation.

Kapha individuals, characterized by their grounded and stable nature, may find it difficult to disengage from their daily routines. Their tendency towards sluggishness requires an approach that encourages lightness and activity. A brisk walk or some light stretching can help to stimulate the body and prepare it for rest. Avoid heavy meals before bed; instead, opt for a light and easily digestible meal several hours before sleeping. Since Kapha types might experience a sluggishness that hinders their transition to sleep, lighter forms of exercise and gentle stimulation may be beneficial to create a feeling of lightness rather than heaviness. This could even include a stimulating, but not overwhelming, conversation with a friend. For Kaphas, maintaining a clean and orderly sleep environment also contributes to a peaceful night's rest. Their constitution thrives on routine, so maintaining a consistent bedtime is crucial.

Regardless of your dosha type, several universal practices contribute to a peaceful and restorative sleep. Aromatherapy plays a significant role. The use of essential oils like lavender, chamomile, sandalwood, and rose can create a calming atmosphere and promote relaxation. These oils can be diffused into the air, added to a warm bath, or applied topically to the pulse points. Furthermore, the practice of mindful meditation, even for just 10-15 minutes before bed, can significantly reduce stress and anxiety, paving the way for a more restful sleep. Focusing on the breath, and observing thoughts and sensations without judgment, can help quiet the mind and prepare it for sleep.

Creating a consistent bedtime routine is also essential. This could include a warm bath or shower, gentle stretches, reading a book, or listening to relaxing music. Consistency reinforces the body's natural circadian rhythm, signaling to the brain that it's time to wind down and prepare for sleep. Avoid caffeine and alcohol in the evening, as these substances can interfere with sleep quality. Similarly, avoid large meals or heavy snacks close to bedtime, as digestion can disrupt sleep. A light, easily digestible snack like a small bowl of warm milk with a pinch of turmeric or a small handful of almonds can be beneficial, especially for those who experience nighttime hunger.

The bedroom environment plays a crucial role in promoting restful sleep. Maintain a cool, dark, and quiet environment. Make sure your bedroom is clean and well-ventilated. A comfortable mattress and pillows are also essential for ensuring proper support and alignment. Consider using blackout curtains or an eye mask to block out light, and earplugs to minimize noise. These seemingly small details can significantly improve the quality of your sleep. Additionally, investing in high-quality bedding made from natural materials like cotton or linen can further contribute to a more comfortable and restful sleep environment.

Beyond these practical suggestions, fostering a sense of mental and emotional calm is paramount for promoting restorative sleep. Before bed, take some time to reflect on the day's events and express gratitude for the positive experiences. Journaling can be a valuable tool for processing emotions and releasing any lingering tension or anxiety. Practicing forgiveness, both of oneself and others, can contribute significantly to mental peace and clarity, preparing you for a more tranquil night's sleep. A conscious effort to let go of worries and concerns is crucial. Consider utilizing mindfulness techniques to detach from stressful thoughts and focus instead on the present moment. Engage in practices that promote a sense of gratitude and appreciation, acknowledging the good things in your life.

Ayurveda emphasizes the holistic nature of health, underscoring the interconnectedness of mind, body, and spirit. A restful sleep is not merely a physical process; it's a time of deep rejuvenation and restoration. By incorporating the principles of Sandhya Dinacharya into your evening routine, you are not only preparing your body for rest but also nurturing your mind and spirit. This leads to improved well-being, increased energy levels, and enhanced resilience to stress. Remember that consistency is key. By making these practices a regular part of your evening routine, you'll gradually notice a significant positive shift in your sleep quality and overall health. Embrace the beauty of Ayurveda's holistic approach and cultivate an evening routine that

harmonizes with your unique constitution, leading you to a deeper, more restorative, and ultimately healthier sleep. This commitment to a well-structured evening routine will not only improve your sleep but also profoundly enhance the quality of your life. The power of a good night's rest shouldn't be underestimated. It is the foundation upon which a healthy and balanced life is built.

Importance of Sleep Hygiene in Ayurvedic Practice

Building upon the principles of Sandhya Dinacharya, we now turn our attention to the critical role of sleep hygiene within the Ayurvedic framework. In Ayurveda, sleep, or *nidra*, is considered one of the three pillars of health, alongside proper diet and lifestyle. The quality of your sleep directly impacts your physical and mental well-being, influencing everything from your digestive strength and immune function to your cognitive acuity and emotional stability. A consistent and well-structured sleep routine, tailored to your individual dosha, is paramount for maintaining balance and promoting optimal health.

The Ayurvedic perspective on sleep goes beyond simply achieving a certain number of hours of rest. It emphasizes the importance of *quality* sleep, a state of deep, restful slumber where the body and mind can fully rejuvenate. This deep rest is crucial for the body to perform its vital processes, including tissue repair, hormone regulation, and waste elimination. Disrupted sleep, on the other hand, can lead to an imbalance of the doshas, resulting in a range of physical and mental health issues, including decreased immunity, digestive problems, weight gain, hormonal imbalances, anxiety, depression, and cognitive impairment.

Understanding the Doshas and Sleep:

Each dosha has unique sleep patterns and preferences. Understanding these differences is key to crafting a personalized sleep hygiene regimen.

Vata:
Individuals with a predominant Vata dosha tend to have light sleep and may experience difficulty falling asleep or staying asleep. They often wake up frequently during the night and may experience restless legs syndrome. Their sleep is often characterized by restlessness and anxiety. To support better sleep for Vata types, the focus should be on creating a calming and grounding bedtime routine. This might include warm milk with a pinch of nutmeg or cardamom, a gentle massage with warm sesame oil, and calming activities like reading a book or listening to soothing music before bed. The bedroom should be warm, dark, and quiet. Avoiding excessive caffeine and stimulating activities before bed is crucial.

Pitta:
Pitta individuals generally have a moderate sleep pattern, but they can be prone to insomnia if they are overstressed or overheated. Their sleep can be interrupted by vivid dreams or nightmares. For Pitta types, it's important to establish a regular sleep schedule and create a cooling and calming environment. This may involve practicing
cooling pranayama techniques like
Sheetali
or
Sheetkari breathwork before bed. Light, cool bedding and a cool room temperature are beneficial. A light, easily digestible dinner is recommended to avoid digestive disturbances that could disrupt sleep. Managing stress is crucial for Pitta individuals prone to sleep disturbances. Regular meditation or calming activities like spending time in nature can significantly
improve their sleep quality.

Kapha:
Kapha individuals tend to sleep heavily and for longer periods. However, they may struggle to wake up early or feel sluggish and groggy throughout the day if they sleep for excessively long periods. For Kapha individuals, it's

essential to establish a regular sleep schedule and focus on lighter, more energizing activities before bed. Avoid heavy, rich foods, particularly close to bedtime. Engaging in light exercise, such as a gentle walk, in the late afternoon can be helpful in promoting a better night's rest. A lighter, brighter room may be preferred to help them wake up feeling more refreshed. Stimulating activities, such as listening to upbeat music or reading an engaging book, can be beneficial in preparing for sleep, provided they don't lead to overstimulation.

Creating a Personalized Sleep Hygiene Routine:

Regardless of your predominant dosha, incorporating the following principles into your daily and evening routine will enhance your sleep quality:

Establish a Regular Sleep Schedule:
Go to bed and wake up at roughly the same time every day, even on weekends, to regulate your body's natural sleep-wake cycle. Consistency is key to establishing a healthy sleep rhythm. This is
particularly important for Vata types prone to inconsistent sleep patterns.

Create a Relaxing Bedtime Routine:
Wind down at least an hour before bedtime. Engage in calming activities such as reading a book, taking a warm bath, listening to soothing music, or practicing gentle yoga or meditation. Avoid
stimulating activities like watching television or using electronic devices close to bedtime. The light emitted from screens interferes with melatonin production, making it difficult to fall asleep.

Optimize Your Sleep Environment:
Ensure your bedroom is dark, quiet, and cool. Invest in comfortable bedding and a supportive mattress. A room that is too bright, noisy, or hot can disrupt sleep. Consider using aromatherapy with calming essential oils such as lavender or chamomile. These gentle aromas can promote relaxation and improve sleep quality.

Pay Attention to Your Diet:
Avoid heavy, rich, or spicy foods close to bedtime. These can cause indigestion and disrupt sleep. A light, easily digestible dinner is
recommended, preferably several hours before bed. For Pitta types, cooling foods and drinks are particularly beneficial. For Vata types, warm, grounding foods are preferable.

Manage Stress:
Stress and anxiety can significantly impair sleep quality. Incorporate stress-reducing techniques into your daily routine, such as yoga, meditation, deep breathing exercises, or spending time in nature. Ayurveda emphasizes the importance of maintaining balance in all aspects of life, and stress management is paramount for optimal sleep.
Consider practicing Ayurvedic techniques like Abhyanga (self-massage) to reduce tension and promote relaxation.

Sunlight Exposure:
Expose yourself to sunlight during the day, particularly in the morning, to regulate your circadian rhythm. Sunlight helps to regulate melatonin production, the hormone that controls your sleep-wake cycle. This is
especially helpful for those who struggle with adjusting their circadian rhythms.

Avoid Caffeine and Alcohol:
These substances can interfere with sleep quality and disrupt your sleep cycle. Limit or avoid their consumption, particularly in the evening.
Caffeine is a stimulant that can keep you awake, while alcohol can disrupt the quality of sleep.

Consider Ayurvedic Herbs and Teas:
Certain Ayurvedic herbs and teas can promote relaxation and improve sleep quality. Consult with an Ayurvedic practitioner for
personalized recommendations. Some herbs known for their calming effects include Ashwagandha, Jatamansi, and

Brahmi. These herbs should be used with caution and under the guidance of a qualified practitioner.

Address Underlying Medical Conditions:
If you consistently experience sleep problems, consult with your doctor or an Ayurvedic practitioner to rule out any underlying medical conditions. Sleep disorders often have root causes that need to be addressed before sleep hygiene practices can fully take effect.

Incorporating these sleep hygiene practices into your daily routine is a significant step towards achieving optimal health and well-being. By prioritizing quality sleep, you are investing in your physical, mental, and emotional health. Remember, consistency is key. Gradually incorporate these practices into your daily life and observe how your sleep quality and overall well-being improve. The path to a healthier, more balanced life begins with the commitment to a good night's sleep. The wisdom of Ayurveda emphasizes that restful sleep is not merely a luxury, but a fundamental necessity for a life of vitality and joy. As you refine your sleep hygiene, pay close attention to how your body responds. This self-awareness is crucial for maintaining balance and tailoring your practices to meet your unique needs. Consider keeping a sleep journal to track your sleep patterns and identify any triggers or patterns that might be impacting your rest. Through careful observation and consistent effort, you can cultivate a deeply restorative sleep that nourishes your body and supports your overall well-being. The journey to better sleep is a personal one, and embracing the principles of Ayurveda will guide you towards a healthier, happier, and more balanced life.

Adapting Your Dinacharya to Your Dosha and Lifestyle

Adapting your Dinacharya to your Dosha and Lifestyle requires a nuanced understanding of your unique constitution and the demands of your daily life. While the foundational principles of Dinacharya remain constant – a structured daily routine that promotes balance – the specific practices and timings need to be personalized to achieve optimal results. A rigid adherence to a prescribed routine, without considering individual needs, can lead to stress and ultimately disrupt the very balance it aims to achieve. The key is to find a harmonious blend of Ayurvedic principles and practical adaptability.

For instance, the ideal wake-up time of Brahma Muhurta (approximately 1.5 hours before sunrise) might be challenging for individuals with demanding jobs or irregular work schedules. While striving for this early rising is beneficial for most, a more realistic approach might involve waking up an hour before sunrise, gradually adjusting the wake-up time as your body adapts. The focus should be on consistency rather than strict adherence to a potentially unattainable ideal.

Similarly, the recommended oil massage (Abhyanga) may need to be adjusted based on the individual's lifestyle. A 15-minute massage might be feasible for some, while others might only manage a 5-minute quick massage on busy days. Even a shorter massage is far more beneficial than none at all. The essential aspect is to incorporate the practice regularly, even if it needs to be adapted to fit a busy schedule. The same flexibility applies to other aspects of the routine, such as meditation, yoga, and pranayama. Instead of aiming for a lengthy session daily, shorter, more frequent sessions might be more sustainable. For example, five minutes of mindful breathing throughout the day can be more effective than a thirty-minute meditation session attempted once a week.

Dosha-specific adjustments are crucial for effective Dinacharya. Vata individuals, prone to dryness and instability, benefit from warm oil massages and a slower-paced routine. They might find it easier to integrate the routine by starting with smaller, manageable chunks and gradually increasing the duration and intensity as their body acclimatizes. Pitta individuals, characterized by a fiery nature, benefit from cooling practices and a more structured routine to prevent overheating. Their Dinacharya should incorporate cooling foods and activities and avoid strenuous exercises during peak sun hours. Kapha individuals, known for their stability and grounded nature, need to incorporate more dynamic activities to prevent stagnation. They might benefit from more rigorous exercise routines and a faster-paced Dinacharya.

The location and environment also influence the effectiveness of the Dinacharya. Practicing yoga in a serene, well-ventilated space is preferable to exercising in a noisy or cluttered environment. Similarly, finding quiet time for meditation amidst the daily hustle and bustle might require adjusting your routine to accommodate quieter periods or using noise-canceling headphones. The crucial aspect is to create a supportive environment that enhances the practice, regardless of the constraints of your living situation.

Seasonal variations significantly affect the effectiveness of Dinacharya. The routine needs to be adapted to the changing climatic conditions. During winter, incorporating more warming practices, such as drinking warm herbal teas and consuming warming spices, is essential for Vata and Kapha types. Similarly, during summer, cooling practices such as incorporating more cooling foods and staying hydrated are crucial for Pitta and Kapha types. Observing the seasonal changes and adjusting the routine accordingly is essential for maintaining balance throughout the year.

Individual preferences and circumstances also play a pivotal role in customizing the Dinacharya. Individuals with health conditions or physical limitations might need to modify the routine to accommodate their specific needs. For instance, individuals with joint pain might need to modify certain yoga poses or opt for gentler forms of exercise. Likewise, individuals with sleep disorders might need to adapt their bedtime routine to address specific challenges. Consulting with an Ayurvedic practitioner is crucial for tailoring the Dinacharya to suit individual circumstances and health conditions.

Sustainability is a key factor in the long-term success of Dinacharya. A routine that is too demanding or difficult to maintain will eventually be abandoned. The key is to start slowly, incorporating one or two practices at a time, and gradually building upon them as your body adapts. Begin with the most essential aspects of the routine, such as maintaining a consistent sleep schedule and incorporating mindful practices like deep breathing. Once these practices become habitual, you can then gradually integrate other elements such as oil massage and yoga.

Accountability also plays a significant role in maintaining a consistent routine. Sharing your goals with a friend or family member, joining a support group, or working with an Ayurvedic practitioner can provide the necessary encouragement and guidance. Tracking your progress and celebrating your successes can reinforce positive habits and increase your motivation. Remember, the aim is to create a sustainable lifestyle that promotes balance and well-being.

In addition to the core practices, consider incorporating other elements into your Dinacharya that resonate with your individual needs and preferences. This could include spending time in nature, listening to calming music, engaging in creative activities, or practicing gratitude. The key is to tailor the routine to your unique preferences and to create a sense of joy and anticipation around the daily practices. It's essential to listen to your body and adjust the routine based on how you feel. If you experience any discomfort, modify the practice or seek guidance from an Ayurvedic professional.

Finally, remember that adapting your Dinacharya is an ongoing process. As your life circumstances change, so too should your routine. Be flexible, patient, and compassionate with yourself. Celebrate your successes, learn from your setbacks, and remain committed to your well-being. The goal is to create a daily routine that is not only effective but also enjoyable and sustainable in the long term, fostering a balanced and harmonious life aligned with your individual needs and the wisdom of Ayurveda. The journey toward optimal health through Dinacharya is a personal one, uniquely tailored to you. Embrace the process, and enjoy the journey towards a healthier, happier you.

Yoga and Pranayama for Each Dosha

Ayurveda recognizes the interconnectedness of body, mind, and spirit, and yoga and pranayama (breathing techniques) are integral to maintaining this balance. Different asanas (yoga postures) and breathing exercises are recommended depending on your dominant dosha, as each dosha has unique energetic characteristics that require specific approaches. This personalized approach helps to harmonize the doshas and promote overall well-being.

For those with a predominantly
Vata
dosha, characterized by air and ether elements, the primary aim of yoga and
pranayama is to ground and stabilize the energy. Vata individuals tend to be prone to anxiety, insomnia, and digestive issues. Therefore, the practice should focus on calming the nervous system and promoting grounding. Gentle, flowing movements are ideal, rather than vigorous or intense practices. Poses that promote stability and strength, such as Tree Pose (Vrksasana), Mountain Pose (Tadasana), and Chair Pose (Utkatasana), are excellent choices. These poses help to anchor the Vata energy and prevent excessive movement.

Incorporating grounding asanas is vital. These poses connect you to the earth, calming the often flighty Vata energy. Think of poses that involve a wide, stable base, like Warrior II (Virabhadrasana II). Holding these poses, even for short durations, promotes stability and a sense of centeredness. Furthermore, including forward folds like Seated Forward Bend (Paschimottanasana) gently stretches and calms the nervous system. Remember to practice these poses with a slow, deliberate approach, avoiding jerky movements.

Pranayama for Vata should emphasize slow, deep, and rhythmic breathing. Dirga Pranayama (three-part breath) is particularly beneficial. This technique involves inhaling deeply into the abdomen, then the chest, and finally the collarbones, followed by a slow, controlled exhalation. This rhythmic breathing helps to regulate the breath and calm the mind. Nadi Shodhana Pranayama (alternate nostril breathing) is another excellent practice to balance the energies and calm the nervous system. It's vital to ensure the practice remains gentle; avoid forceful breathing, which could further aggravate Vata imbalance. Regular practice, even for just 10-15 minutes daily, can significantly improve sleep, reduce anxiety, and enhance overall well-being.

Individuals with a predominantly
Pitta
dosha, characterized by fire and water elements, are often energetic, ambitious, and intelligent. However, they can also be prone to
irritability, anger, and inflammation. Yoga and pranayama for Pitta should focus on cooling and calming the fiery energy. Cooling poses such as Triangle Pose (Trikonasana), Half Moon Pose (Ardha Chandrasana), and Extended Side Angle Pose (Utthita Parsvakonasana) are beneficial. These poses help to lengthen the spine and stretch the sides of the body, promoting a feeling of coolness and relaxation. Backbends should be practiced with caution, as they could potentially increase Pitta's fiery nature. It's best to opt for gentler backbends, only if they feel comfortable, and to avoid intense stretches.

Cooling pranayama practices are particularly beneficial for Pitta. Sheetali Pranayama (cooling breath) involves curling the tongue and inhaling through the mouth, followed by exhaling through the nose. This technique helps to cool the body and calm the mind. Shitali Pranayama can be a powerful tool, especially during hot weather or when experiencing feelings of irritation or anger. It's important to remember to maintain a relaxed and controlled breathing pattern. Sitapali Pranayama is a variation for those unable to curl their tongues, in which they inhale through the pursed lips. These techniques provide a direct cooling effect, helping to reduce the intensity of Pitta.

For
Kapha
dosha, characterized by earth and water elements, the focus of yoga and pranayama should be on energizing and stimulating the body. Kapha individuals are often calm, grounded, and stable, but they can also be prone to sluggishness, weight gain, and respiratory issues. Therefore, the practice should focus on increasing energy levels and promoting detoxification. Energizing poses such as Sun Salutations (Surya Namaskar), Warrior II (Virabhadrasana II), and Triangle Pose (Trikonasana) are ideal. These poses increase circulation, invigorate the body, and help to remove stagnant energy. Kapha individuals may benefit from more vigorous practice styles, but should avoid overdoing it, listening to their bodies and avoiding pushing too hard.

Pranayama for Kapha should focus on increasing energy and improving circulation. Kapalabhati Pranayama (skull shining breath) involves forceful exhalations, followed by passive inhalations. This technique helps to clear the respiratory system and increase energy levels, but it should be done cautiously and with awareness. Bhastrika Pranayama (bellows breath) is another vigorous technique that can help boost energy, but it's important to pay attention to your physical sensations and avoid strain. Alternatively, Ujjayi Pranayama (victorious breath) can create a gentle warmth and energy in the body without being overly stimulating.

Regardless of your dominant dosha, remember that consistency is key. Even a short daily practice of yoga and pranayama can have significant benefits. Start slowly, listen to your body, and gradually increase the intensity and duration of your practice. It is also important to find a style of yoga that suits your personality and preferences. Some styles, such as Hatha Yoga, are generally more gentle and suitable for all doshas, while others, like Vinyasa Yoga, are more vigorous and may be better suited for Kapha individuals.

Remember that the practice of yoga and pranayama is not a race, but a journey of self-discovery and self-healing. It's recommended to consult with a qualified yoga instructor or Ayurvedic practitioner to create a personalized practice that meets your individual needs and goals, especially if you have any health conditions or pre-existing injuries. They can guide you towards the right poses and breathing exercises, ensuring you are practicing safely and effectively. The goal is to find a practice that supports your unique constitution and helps you to achieve a state of balance and harmony. The benefits extend beyond physical health, touching upon mental clarity, emotional stability, and a deeper connection with your inner self. Through mindful practice, you can unlock the transformative power of Ayurveda and yoga to enhance your overall well-being.

Walking Swimming and More

Beyond the structured practice of yoga and pranayama, Ayurveda embraces a broader spectrum of physical activity to promote balance and well-being. While yoga forms the cornerstone of Ayurvedic exercise, incorporating other forms of movement can significantly enhance your overall health and vitality. The key, as always, lies in selecting activities that harmonize with your unique doshic constitution. Let's delve into some readily accessible and beneficial options.

Walking, often underestimated, is a profoundly effective form of exercise, easily adaptable to individual needs and preferences. For Vata individuals, prone to dryness and instability, a brisk walk can be incredibly grounding. However, it's essential to avoid overexertion, which can exacerbate Vata's tendency towards anxiety and exhaustion. A moderate pace, preferably in nature amidst calming surroundings, is ideal. The rhythmic movement helps to stabilize Vata energy, promoting a sense of calm and centeredness. Incorporating walks into your daily routine, even short 15-20 minute strolls, can significantly contribute to overall well-being. Remember to choose comfortable, supportive footwear to prevent jarring the joints. Consider walking barefoot on grass or sand whenever possible to further ground yourself and enhance sensory awareness. The grounding properties of earth will help balance the lightness and airy nature of Vata.

Pitta individuals, characterized by their fiery and energetic nature, often benefit from activities that help to cool and calm the system. While walking is suitable, they should opt for a more moderate pace than Vata types, avoiding strenuous exertion in intense heat. Early morning or late evening walks, when the sun is less intense, are preferable. The focus should be on maintaining a consistent rhythm without pushing themselves too hard. After a walk, Pitta individuals will find that cooling activities, such as a refreshing shower or a cool drink of water, will be beneficial.

For Kapha individuals, known for their grounded and stable nature, regular walking is crucial to counter their tendency towards sluggishness. A brisk walk, particularly in the morning to stimulate their metabolism, can help to boost energy levels and improve circulation. They tend to enjoy longer walks and may find a more vigorous pace suits their constitution. However, they need to be mindful not to overdo it; listening to their body and adjusting the intensity and duration is crucial to prevent becoming fatigued or overheated. Walking in a park or lively setting can also provide the mental stimulation a Kapha individual may need to avoid stagnation.

Swimming offers a unique set of benefits, adaptable to all three doshas, albeit with subtle adjustments. For Vata, the rhythmic and fluid nature of swimming provides a calming and balancing effect. The constant movement helps to ground the Vata energy, reducing anxiety and promoting relaxation. However, Vata types should avoid cold water, opting for warmer pools or swimming in the summer months.

Pitta individuals, with their naturally fiery constitution, may find swimming particularly beneficial for cooling the body and reducing excess heat. The water's coolness helps to balance Pitta's tendency towards inflammation and irritability. They should choose a moderate pace and avoid overly competitive or strenuous swimming, focusing on rhythmic, gentle movements.

Kapha individuals may find the gentle resistance of the water ideal for stimulating their metabolism and promoting circulation. They can enjoy longer swimming sessions, focusing on maintaining a consistent rhythm and pacing themselves to avoid exhaustion. However, choosing a brisk pace will be more beneficial for Kapha types than a slower one.

Beyond walking and swimming, a multitude of other exercises can effectively complement an Ayurvedic lifestyle. Cycling, a low-impact activity, suits all doshas. For Vata, the rhythmic pedaling provides grounding stability; for Pitta, it offers a cooling cardiovascular workout; and for Kapha, it promotes circulation and energy expenditure. Similarly, dancing, a joyful and expressive form of movement, can be adapted to each dosha. Vata types might benefit from structured, grounding forms of dance, while Pitta could explore more fluid and flowing styles, and Kapha might enjoy more energetic, rhythmic movement.

Tai chi, a gentle martial art, is a fantastic option for cultivating balance and promoting tranquility. Its slow, deliberate movements promote mindfulness and coordination, making it particularly suitable for Vata and Pitta individuals. Kapha individuals can also benefit from its grounding and gentle stretching. Qi gong, another mindful movement practice, shares similar benefits, focusing on the flow of energy within the body. Both tai chi and Qi gong are excellent stress reducers, promoting relaxation and helping to harmonize the mind and body. These practices will allow for better balance and overall well-being.

Gardening, while often not considered a strenuous exercise, can significantly impact physical and mental health. The gentle stretching, bending, and lifting involved provide a gentle workout, while the connection with nature promotes relaxation and stress reduction. The grounding nature of working with the earth is particularly beneficial for Vata individuals, while the mindful attention to detail helps to calm Pitta. For Kapha, gardening can provide a healthy outlet for energy and creativity.

The key to selecting the appropriate exercise is understanding your unique doshic constitution and selecting activities that harmonize with your energetic profile. Avoid activities that exacerbate your doshic imbalances, focusing instead on practices that nurture balance and promote overall well-being. Remember that the ideal exercise routine is a personalized one, tailored to your specific needs and preferences. Start slowly, gradually increasing intensity and duration as your fitness improves. Always listen to your body and stop if you experience pain or discomfort.

Furthermore, the time of day when you exercise also plays a significant role in optimizing its benefits. For example, morning exercises are often recommended for Kapha individuals to jumpstart their metabolism. Late afternoons or early evenings may be more suitable for Vata individuals to help them wind down after a day's activities. Pitta individuals should try to avoid exercising during the hottest parts of the day.

The integration of exercise into your daily routine is paramount to maintain a state of balance and health, but it is also essential to listen to your body and to consult with a healthcare professional before starting any new exercise regime. Remember that the goal is not to push yourself to the limits but to engage in activities that bring you joy, promote harmony, and help you cultivate a deeper connection with yourself. The path to holistic wellness in Ayurveda is paved with mindful movement, tailored to your individual needs and constitution. This holistic approach to fitness will enhance your quality of life and allow for a better sense of balance and overall wellness.

The Importance of mindful movement

Mindful movement transcends the mere physical act of exercise; it's a profound practice that cultivates a harmonious connection between body and mind. In Ayurveda, this connection is vital, as imbalances in either sphere inevitably affect the other. When we move mindfully, we become acutely aware of our body's sensations, our breath, and the subtle energies flowing within us. This awareness allows us to adjust our movements, preventing strain and promoting a sense of ease and fluidity. It's not about striving for perfection or achieving peak physical condition; instead, it's about cultivating a gentle, respectful relationship with our physical selves.

Consider, for instance, the simple act of walking. Most of us rush through our daily walks, our minds preoccupied with thoughts of work, errands, or other commitments. Mindful walking, however, transforms this mundane activity into a meditative practice. Pay attention to the sensation of your feet making contact with the ground, the rhythm of your breath, and the movement of your body. Notice the subtle shifts in your posture, the way your muscles engage and release. Feel the gentle sway of your arms, the expansion of your chest as you inhale, and the gentle contraction as you exhale. Engage all your senses: observe the sights, sounds, and smells around you. By bringing your awareness to the present moment, you transform a simple walk into a restorative and rejuvenating experience.

This principle of mindful awareness can be applied to any form of movement. Whether you're practicing yoga, engaging in gardening, dancing, swimming, or simply doing household chores, the focus should always be on cultivating a present-moment awareness. Feel the subtle nuances of each movement, paying attention to your breath and the sensations in your body. Avoid pushing yourself too hard; instead, let your movements be guided by your breath and your body's natural rhythm. If you feel any pain or discomfort, stop and adjust your posture or the intensity of the movement. Listen to your body's wisdom; it is always communicating with you, providing valuable feedback on your physical and energetic state.

For those with a predominantly Vata constitution, mindful movement should emphasize gentle, flowing movements that promote grounding and stability. Avoid strenuous activities or rapid, jerky motions that might further exacerbate the Vata's tendency towards instability. Gentle forms of yoga like Hatha yoga, restorative yoga, and even mindful walking are ideal choices. These practices help to calm the nervous system and promote a sense of centeredness. Furthermore, incorporating grounding activities like Tai Chi or Qigong can help to further anchor Vata energy, preventing it from becoming scattered and erratic. Regular, consistent practice is key, even if it's just for a few minutes each day. Consistency is more important than intensity.

Individuals with a predominantly Pitta constitution benefit from mindful movement that helps to cool and calm the fiery Pitta energy. Activities that promote a sense of coolness and relaxation are ideal. Swimming, particularly in cool water, can be incredibly beneficial. Likewise, gentle forms of yoga, such as Yin yoga or restorative yoga, can help to counteract the intensity of Pitta energy. Avoid overly strenuous activities or competitive sports that might overheat the body and further aggravate the Pitta dosha. Remember that the goal is to balance and harmonize the Pitta energy, not to push it to its limits. Regular breaks throughout your day, incorporating mindful breathing exercises, can also help to cool down the body and prevent excessive heat build-up.

For those with a predominantly Kapha constitution, mindful movement should focus on stimulating and energizing the body and mind. Kapha individuals often benefit from more vigorous forms of exercise that help to break up stagnation and promote a sense of lightness. Cardiovascular exercise like brisk walking, jogging, cycling, or dancing can be highly beneficial. Yoga styles that incorporate more dynamic movements, such as Ashtanga or Vinyasa yoga, can also be helpful. The key is to find activities that are stimulating and engaging without being overly strenuous. Regular movement is essential to counter the Kapha dosha's tendency towards sluggishness and inertia. Choosing activities you enjoy is crucial for long-term adherence, ensuring you maintain a consistent practice.

Regardless of your predominant dosha, incorporating mindful movement into your daily routine offers numerous benefits. It not only strengthens your physical body but also improves your mental clarity, reduces stress, enhances your mood, and promotes a deeper sense of self-awareness. It's a holistic practice that integrates the mind, body, and spirit, bringing you into closer alignment with your inner self. It's about cultivating a relationship with your body that is characterized by respect, gentleness, and compassion. It's about tuning into the subtle signals that your body sends and responding accordingly.

To further enhance the benefits of mindful movement, consider incorporating specific Ayurvedic practices. For example, Abhyanga, the Ayurvedic practice of self-massage with warm, medicated oils, can help to prepare the body for physical activity by lubricating the joints and relaxing the muscles. After your mindful movement session, practicing

Shatkarmas, or Ayurvedic cleansing techniques, such as Jala Neti (nasal cleansing with saline water) or Kunjal (gentle gastric lavage), can help to eliminate toxins and promote deeper relaxation.

Furthermore, integrating the principles of Dinacharya, the Ayurvedic daily routine, into your day can significantly enhance the benefits of mindful movement. By incorporating regular exercise into your daily schedule at a consistent time, you are laying the foundation for a more balanced and harmonious lifestyle. This consistency promotes the body's ability to regulate its internal systems, maximizing the benefits of your chosen form of mindful movement. Remember to listen to your body, adjusting the intensity and duration of your practice as needed. Don't push yourself beyond your limits; instead, focus on cultivating a sustainable and enjoyable practice that nourishes both your body and your mind.

Beyond the formal practice of mindful movement, consider infusing movement into your daily life. Take the stairs instead of the elevator. Walk or cycle instead of driving short distances. Engage in activities that require physical exertion, such as gardening, cleaning, or household chores. By incorporating movement into your everyday routine, you create a lifestyle that promotes health and well-being, rather than viewing exercise as a separate, scheduled activity. This subtle shift in perspective transforms movement from a chore into a vital aspect of a holistic, balanced life.

Ultimately, the key to successful integration of mindful movement lies in finding activities you genuinely enjoy. If you find an activity tedious or unpleasant, you're less likely to stick with it. Experiment with different forms of movement until you find what resonates with you and your body's unique needs. Whether it's yoga, dance, swimming, gardening, or simply taking a mindful walk in nature, the goal is to find activities that bring you joy, promote a sense of ease and balance, and foster a deeper connection between your body and mind. This mindful approach will not only enhance your physical health but also cultivate a greater sense of peace, well-being, and harmony within yourself. Remember that the journey toward optimal health is a personal one, and the path of mindful movement offers a profound and transformative way to connect with your body and unlock your full potential for vibrant well-being. The consistent practice of mindful movement, tailored to your individual dosha and preferences, will become a cornerstone of your Ayurvedic journey towards a healthier, more balanced, and fulfilling life.

Creating a personalized exercise plan

Creating a personalized exercise plan is crucial for achieving lasting wellness within the Ayurvedic framework. It's not simply about choosing a workout regimen; it's about understanding your unique constitution – your dosha – and selecting activities that support its inherent qualities while mitigating any potential imbalances. Remember, the goal isn't to exhaust yourself but to cultivate a harmonious relationship with your body, fostering strength, flexibility, and vitality.

The first step is to determine your predominant dosha. If you haven't already done so using the Dosha Wheel provided earlier in the book, take some time to reflect on your physical and mental characteristics. Do you tend to be energetic and quick-moving (Vata), fiery and ambitious (Pitta), or grounded and steady (Kapha)? Understanding your primary dosha provides a roadmap for choosing exercises that naturally align with your constitution.

For individuals with a predominantly
Vata
dosha,
characterized by air and ether elements, the emphasis should be on grounding and stabilizing practices. Vigorous, high-impact exercises can exacerbate Vata's tendency toward anxiety and restlessness. Instead, opt for gentle, rhythmic activities that promote stability and calmness. Yoga styles like Hatha or restorative yoga, which focus on slower movements and longer holds, are particularly beneficial. Tai chi and Qi gong, with their flowing movements and meditative aspects, are also excellent choices. Incorporating walking in nature, especially in calm, soothing environments, can be incredibly restorative. Avoid overly strenuous exercises or activities that lead to excessive

sweating or breathlessness. Aim for consistency over intensity. Regular, moderate exercise is more effective than sporadic bursts of high-intensity activity.

Those with a **Pitta** dosha, dominated by fire and water, possess energetic and dynamic qualities. Pitta individuals thrive on challenge and often excel in competitive sports. However, their fiery nature makes them prone to overheating and burnout. Therefore, it's crucial to choose exercises that allow for a balance of intensity and cooling. Activities like swimming, cycling, and brisk walking are excellent options, offering a moderate level of exertion without overstimulating the body. Yoga styles like Vinyasa or Ashtanga, with their flowing sequences, can be beneficial but should be approached with caution, ensuring ample rest and hydration. Avoid intense, competitive activities in hot and humid conditions, which can exacerbate Pitta's already fiery nature. Focus on mindful movement, paying close attention to your body's signals and slowing down when needed. Remember that regular breaks and cooling practices are vital to avoid overheating and maintaining equilibrium.

Individuals with a **Kapha** dosha, characterized by earth and water, are typically strong and stable, but they can be prone to sluggishness and weight gain if they are not physically active. Kapha individuals benefit from invigorating exercises that stimulate circulation and promote lightness. Activities like brisk walking, jogging, swimming, and dancing are excellent choices. These activities help to increase metabolism and reduce the build-up of excess Kapha. Yoga styles like Ashtanga or power yoga, which are more vigorous and stimulating, can also be beneficial. However, it's essential to avoid overly sedentary activities, and to ensure that exercise is a consistent part of your daily or weekly routine. The key for Kapha is to build up a sweat, and to consistently maintain regular exercise. Avoid exercises that are too slow or gentle, which might not be stimulating enough to counteract their tendency towards sluggishness.

Beyond the doshic considerations, your personal preferences and physical limitations are equally crucial. Choose activities you genuinely enjoy, making exercise a pleasurable part of your life rather than a dreaded chore. If you dislike running, don't force yourself; explore other options like dancing, hiking, or cycling. Consider any physical limitations or injuries; don't push your body beyond its comfortable limits. If you have any pre-existing health conditions, consult with your doctor or a qualified physical therapist before starting a new exercise program.

A well-structured Ayurvedic exercise plan should encompass various elements:

Warm-up:
Begin each exercise session with 5-10 minutes of gentle movements like stretching or light cardio to prepare your body for more intense activity. This helps to increase blood flow, improve flexibility, and reduce the risk of injury.

Main activity:
Choose an activity suitable for your dosha and preferences. Allocate 30-60 minutes to this part of your session. Pay attention to your body's signals; if you feel any pain or discomfort, stop immediately.

Cool-down:
Conclude your session with 5-10 minutes of gentle stretching or relaxation techniques like deep breathing or meditation. This helps to lower your heart rate, promote muscle recovery, and enhance the overall sense of calm.

Remember, consistency is key. Aim for regular exercise, even if it's just for a short period, rather than infrequent intense sessions. Start slowly and gradually increase the duration and intensity of your workouts as your fitness level improves. Listen to your body's signals and adjust your routine accordingly.

Incorporating Ayurvedic principles into your exercise regimen extends beyond the type of activity you choose. It also involves considering the time of day, the season, and your overall energy levels. For example, early mornings are generally considered the best time to exercise for most doshas, as the environment is typically cooler and calmer. However, Kapha individuals might prefer later morning or early afternoon when they have more energy. During the hotter summer months, opt for activities that keep you cool, such as swimming or yoga in an air-conditioned space.

To further personalize your exercise plan, consider keeping a journal to track your workouts, monitor your progress, and make necessary adjustments. Note your energy levels before and after each exercise session, the type of activity, the duration, and any physical sensations. This record can help you identify what works best for your body and adjust your plan accordingly.

Beyond formal exercise, incorporate movement into your daily routine. Take the stairs instead of the elevator, walk or cycle instead of driving short distances, and get up and move around every 30 minutes if you have a sedentary job. These small changes can significantly impact your overall fitness and well-being.

Remember, the ultimate goal of an Ayurvedic exercise plan is not to achieve a specific body shape or attain a certain level of fitness; it's to cultivate a harmonious relationship with your body, fostering strength, flexibility, and vitality. It's about finding activities that bring you joy, promote balance, and nourish your physical and mental well-being.

Embrace this mindful approach to movement, and you will discover the transformative power of exercise within the context of Ayurvedic living. The journey towards a healthier, more balanced you begins with a single step, a single breath, a single mindful movement. And remember, consistency and self-compassion are crucial allies on this path.

Maintaining Equilibrium

The practice of exercise, or *vyayama* in Sanskrit, holds a central place within the Ayurvedic system. It's not merely about physical exertion; it's a vital tool for maintaining the delicate equilibrium of the three doshas – Vata, Pitta, and Kapha – and preventing the onset of disease. Regular physical activity, tailored to your individual doshic constitution, can significantly enhance your overall health and well-being, promoting strength, flexibility, and a balanced state of mind.

Understanding how each dosha responds to different types of exercise is critical for creating a personalized regimen. Ignoring this crucial element can lead to imbalances and even exacerbate existing health concerns. For instance, vigorous, high-impact exercise, while beneficial for some, could be detrimental to others. The key lies in aligning your exercise routine with your unique doshic nature, fostering a harmonious relationship between your body and mind.

Vata Dosha and Exercise:

Individuals with a predominantly Vata constitution are characterized by their lightness, dryness, and a tendency towards anxiety. Their energy is often scattered and erratic. Therefore, Vata types benefit from exercise routines that are gentle, grounding, and rhythmic. Avoid strenuous activities that can further deplete their energy and lead to exhaustion.

Ideal exercises for Vatas include:

Yoga:
Gentle Hatha yoga, focusing on restorative postures and breathwork (pranayama), is particularly beneficial.

Poses that promote stability and grounding, such as tree pose (Vrksasana) and mountain pose (Tadasana), are excellent choices. Avoid fast-paced, vigorous styles of yoga like Ashtanga or Vinyasa.

Walking:
A moderate-paced walk in nature is a wonderful way for Vatas to connect with the earth and calm their nervous system. The rhythmic movement helps to stabilize their energy and promote a sense of calm.

Swimming:
The gentle resistance of water can be very soothing for Vata's tendency towards dryness and instability.

Dancing:
Slow, graceful dances like ballroom or folk dancing can be both enjoyable and beneficial, promoting coordination and grounding.

Tai Chi and Qigong:
These gentle, flowing movement practices help to cultivate inner peace and balance the nervous system, ideal for calming Vata's restless energy.

It's crucial for Vatas to avoid intense cardio workouts, competitive sports, and activities that lead to excessive sweating or dehydration, which can exacerbate their already dry constitution. Regularity is key; short, frequent sessions are preferable to long, strenuous ones. It's also essential to incorporate relaxation techniques, such as meditation or deep breathing exercises, into their daily routine to further enhance balance and prevent burnout. Remember, the goal is to gently nurture and stabilize the Vata energy, not deplete it.

Pitta Dosha and Exercise:

Pitta individuals are characterized by their fiery, passionate nature and a tendency towards intensity. They are often driven and ambitious, but this can lead to stress and burnout if not managed effectively. Pitta types need exercise that helps them release excess heat and energy while avoiding overexertion.

Suitable exercises for Pittas include:

Yoga:
Vinyasa or Ashtanga yoga, when practiced with moderation, can be beneficial in releasing excess heat and building strength. However, it's essential to avoid pushing oneself too hard and to incorporate plenty of cooling practices like savasana (corpse pose).

Swimming:
Swimming is an excellent choice as it cools the body and provides a full-body workout without excessive exertion.

Cycling:
Moderate cycling can be a good way to release pent-up energy while enjoying the outdoors.

Martial arts (with modifications):
Certain martial arts styles, like Tai Chi Chuan, can be adapted to suit Pitta's constitution. Focus on gentle movements and breathing techniques to avoid overheating and overstimulation.

Team sports (with moderation):
Team sports can be enjoyable for Pittas, but it's important to avoid becoming overly competitive and to listen to the body's signals.

Exercises to avoid for Pittas include those that generate excessive heat, such as hot yoga, intense weightlifting, and prolonged exposure to intense sunlight. Regular cool showers and hydrating fluids can help to mitigate excess heat generated during exercise. It's important for Pittas to cultivate a sense of balance and avoid pushing themselves to the point of exhaustion. Regular mindful breaks and prioritizing rest are also crucial to maintain balance.

Kapha Dosha and Exercise:

Kapha individuals possess a strong, stable constitution, but they can also be prone to sluggishness and weight gain if they don't engage in regular exercise. They need activities that stimulate their metabolism and promote movement and flexibility.

Beneficial exercises for Kaphas include:

Yoga:
More vigorous styles of yoga, such as Ashtanga or Power Yoga, can be beneficial in stimulating circulation and building strength. However, it's crucial to avoid overexertion. Incorporating twists and dynamic poses is helpful in stimulating the digestive system and promoting detoxification.

Cardiovascular exercise:
Activities like brisk walking, running, or cycling can help to boost metabolism and burn calories, effectively counteracting Kapha's tendency towards weight gain.

Aerobics:
Higher intensity aerobic activities, like Zumba or step aerobics, can be energizing and fun for Kaphas, promoting movement and improving cardiovascular health.

Dancing:
Energetic and rhythmic dances, such as hip-hop or salsa, are excellent ways for Kaphas to release energy and boost their mood.

Team sports:
Team sports can be beneficial in promoting social interaction and encouraging a more active lifestyle.

Kaphas should avoid prolonged periods of inactivity and overly sedentary lifestyles. Maintaining a regular exercise routine is crucial for preventing sluggishness and weight gain. However, they need to be mindful of overdoing it, as their robust constitution can sometimes mask fatigue signals. Listen to your body's signals and avoid pushing through exhaustion. Incorporating stimulating activities and maintaining a balanced lifestyle is key to promoting overall health and vitality.

Exercise and Seasonal Adjustments:

It's also essential to adjust your exercise routine according to the changing seasons. During the hotter months (Pitta season), opt for cooler activities and avoid intense workouts during the peak heat. In the colder months (Kapha season), choose exercises that generate warmth and invigorate the body. The Vata season (autumn/winter) calls for gentle, grounding exercises that help to conserve energy and maintain warmth.

Remember, finding the right balance is key. Experiment with different activities, listen to your body, and adjust your routine as needed. The goal is to create an exercise regimen that is enjoyable, sustainable, and helps you maintain the equilibrium of your dosha, leading to a more balanced, healthy, and vibrant life. The journey to a healthy body and mind through exercise is a personal one, requiring self-awareness, patience, and a deep understanding of your individual dosha's needs. Don't be afraid to seek guidance from an Ayurvedic practitioner for personalized recommendations. They can help you tailor your exercise regimen to your unique constitution and ensure that your workouts support your overall health and well-being. The path towards holistic health is paved with mindful choices, including a personalized approach to exercise that harmonizes with your unique constitution and promotes balance within your body and mind. This integrated approach, blending the wisdom of Ayurveda with the benefits of physical activity, is a powerful catalyst for lasting well-being. By understanding your doshic type and choosing activities that support your individual needs, you unlock the potential for a more balanced, vibrant, and fulfilling life. This attentive, personalized approach to exercise is not just about physical fitness; it's about cultivating a harmonious relationship with your body, enhancing your energy levels, and fostering a profound sense of inner peace.

Ayurvedic Techniques for Stress Reduction

Ayurveda, with its holistic approach to health, offers a wealth of techniques for effectively managing stress. Unlike many modern approaches that focus solely on symptom relief, Ayurveda addresses the root cause of stress by
considering the individual's unique constitution (dosha), lifestyle, and environmental factors. This multifaceted approach involves a combination of lifestyle adjustments, dietary modifications, herbal remedies, and mind-body practices.

One of the cornerstone techniques is the practice of meditation, specifically
dhyana
in Ayurveda. This isn't just about clearing your mind; it's about cultivating a state of deep inner peace and awareness. Different styles of
meditation resonate with different doshas. For example, individuals with a Vata dosha, characterized by their airy and flighty nature, might find grounding meditations, involving visualization of the earth element, particularly beneficial. These might include focusing on the sensation of the breath against the skin, or visualizing roots growing down into the earth, drawing stability and calmness. Pitta individuals, known for their fiery and intense nature, might find cooling and calming meditations, incorporating imagery of water or cooler environments, more soothing. Guided meditations with gentle, rhythmic sounds can be particularly effective. Finally, Kapha individuals, typically grounded and stable, could benefit from meditations that encourage lightness and movement, such as walking meditations or visualizations that involve floating or soaring. The key is to find a style that feels naturally compatible with your constitution. Even short, 10-15 minute sessions of daily meditation can significantly reduce stress levels over time.

Aromatherapy plays a significant role in Ayurvedic stress management. Essential oils, carefully chosen based on their properties and the individual's dosha, can help to regulate the nervous system and promote relaxation. For Vata dosha, grounding scents like sandalwood, patchouli, and vetiver are often recommended. These warm, earthy aromas help to stabilize the nervous system and reduce anxiety. For Pitta dosha, cooling and calming scents such as lavender, rose, and jasmine are more appropriate, helping to soothe the fiery nature of this dosha. Kapha individuals might benefit from invigorating and uplifting scents like lemon, eucalyptus, and peppermint, which help to stimulate and clear the mind. These oils can be used in diffusers, applied topically (diluted in a carrier oil), or inhaled directly from the bottle. It's important to always use high-quality, pure essential oils and to follow appropriate safety guidelines.

Herbal remedies provide another powerful tool in the Ayurvedic arsenal for stress management. Many herbs have adaptogenic properties, meaning they help the body adapt to stress and restore balance.
Ashwagandha
(Withania
somnifera) is a well-known adaptogen that has been extensively studied for its stress-reducing effects. It helps to calm the nervous system, reduce cortisol levels, and improve sleep quality.
Brahmi
(Bacopa monnieri) is another valuable herb that supports cognitive function and reduces anxiety. *Tulsi*
(Holy Basil), a revered herb in Ayurveda, has powerful antioxidant and anti-inflammatory properties, supporting the body's ability to cope with stress. These herbs can be consumed as teas, tinctures, or capsules. It's essential to consult with a qualified Ayurvedic practitioner to determine the appropriate dosage and combination of herbs based on individual needs and dosha.

Beyond herbal remedies, lifestyle modifications play a critical role in stress management within Ayurveda. This includes prioritizing sleep, establishing a consistent daily routine (Dinacharya), and engaging in regular physical activity tailored to one's dosha. Insufficient sleep significantly exacerbates stress; hence, Ayurveda emphasizes the importance of 7-8 hours of quality sleep each night. A consistent sleep schedule helps to regulate the body's natural circadian rhythm, promoting better sleep and reducing stress. Regular physical activity helps to release endorphins, natural mood boosters that reduce stress hormones. The type of activity should be chosen based on the individual's dosha: gentle yoga or walking for Vata, moderate swimming or cycling for Pitta, and more vigorous exercise such as brisk walking or team sports for Kapha. Finding activities you enjoy increases your adherence and motivation, maximizing their stress-reducing benefits.

The Ayurvedic concept of *Dinacharya*, or the daily routine, is crucial for stress management. A consistent daily schedule helps to regulate the body's natural rhythms, reducing stress and promoting feelings of stability and control. This routine ideally begins with a calming morning ritual, incorporating activities like tongue scraping, oil pulling, self-massage (Abhyanga), and meditation. These practices help to cleanse the body, soothe the senses, and set a positive tone for the day. The evening routine should focus on winding down before sleep. This might include a warm bath, reading a book, or gentle yoga. Avoiding screen time before bed is also essential. Consistency is key; by creating a predictable and calming daily routine, you can significantly reduce feelings of stress and improve your overall sense of well-being.

Another important aspect of Ayurvedic stress management is the mindful interaction with nature. Spending time outdoors, surrounded by nature, has proven therapeutic effects. The sights, sounds, and smells of nature promote relaxation and reduce feelings of stress and anxiety. Walking barefoot on grass, sitting under a tree, or simply gazing at the sky can have profound calming effects. The connection with nature fosters a sense of groundedness and peace, helping to combat the stresses of modern life.

Finally, creating a personalized stress management plan is crucial for long-term success. This plan should incorporate a combination of techniques that resonate with your individual needs and dosha. It should be a holistic approach, integrating dietary modifications, herbal remedies, lifestyle adjustments, and mind-body practices. Regular self-assessment helps to identify triggers and patterns of stress, allowing for proactive management. Journaling can also be an effective tool for tracking stress levels and progress. Remember to be patient and kind to yourself; implementing these changes takes time and effort. The goal is to integrate these techniques gradually into your life, making sustainable changes that support your overall well-being. Regular consultation with a qualified Ayurvedic practitioner can provide personalized guidance and support throughout this journey, tailoring the approach to your individual needs and helping you navigate challenges along the way. The path to stress reduction in Ayurveda is not a quick fix but a journey towards a more balanced and harmonious life.

Mindfulness and Meditation Practices

Mindfulness and meditation are powerful tools in the Ayurvedic arsenal for stress reduction. They offer a direct pathway to calming the mind and cultivating inner peace, counteracting the effects of chronic stress on the body and mind. Unlike quick fixes, these practices cultivate a deep, lasting sense of equilibrium, essential for maintaining balance in the face of life's challenges. The practice of mindfulness, in particular, involves paying attention to the present moment without judgment. This seemingly simple act has profound effects on the nervous system, gently guiding it away from the fight-or-flight response often triggered by stress.

The Ayurvedic perspective emphasizes the interconnectedness of mind and body. Stress, therefore, isn't simply a mental state; it manifests physically through imbalances in the doshas. Chronic stress can aggravate Vata dosha, leading to anxiety, insomnia, and digestive issues. It can overheat Pitta, resulting in irritability, inflammation, and heartburn. And it can weigh down Kapha, contributing to lethargy, sluggishness, and respiratory problems. Mindfulness and meditation practices act as a balm, helping to restore balance to the doshas by calming the nervous system and promoting a state of inner harmony.

One effective mindfulness technique rooted in Ayurvedic principles is
Pratyahara
, the fifth limb of yoga. Pratyahara translates to "withdrawal of the senses." It's not about
isolation but about consciously directing your attention inward, away from external distractions that fuel the stress response. Practicing Pratyahara involves creating a quiet space, focusing on your breath, and gently turning your

awareness away from sensory inputs – the sounds, sights, smells, tastes, and textures around you. This practice helps to quiet the constant chatter of the mind, allowing for a deeper connection with your inner self. Even a few minutes of Pratyahara each day can significantly reduce stress and improve focus.

Meditation, another cornerstone of stress management in Ayurveda, takes this inward focus further. It involves cultivating a state of deep relaxation and mental clarity. Ayurveda suggests various meditation techniques, each tailored to address specific doshic imbalances. For example, individuals with aggravated Vata dosha might find solace in calming meditations that incorporate slow, rhythmic breathing and gentle visualizations. These practices help to stabilize the nervous system and reduce anxiety. Individuals with Pitta dosha, often prone to overheating, may benefit from cooling meditations, such as focusing on the sensation of cool air entering the nostrils with each inhale. This helps to pacify the fiery Pitta energy and prevent emotional flare-ups. Kapha individuals, prone to stagnation, might find dynamic meditations, those that incorporate movement or chanting, beneficial in energizing the mind and body.

The key to successful meditation in Ayurveda is consistency and patience. It's not about achieving a perfectly still mind; it's about cultivating a regular practice that allows you to gradually develop greater awareness and control over your mental state. Beginners may find it helpful to start with shorter meditation sessions, perhaps five or ten minutes daily, gradually increasing the duration as they become more comfortable. Guided meditations, readily available through apps or online resources, can be a valuable aid for beginners. Finding a quiet, comfortable space free from distractions is also crucial for creating a conducive environment for meditation.

Beyond formal meditation, incorporating mindfulness into everyday activities is equally vital. This can involve practicing mindful eating, savoring each bite and paying attention to the tastes and textures of the food. It can also include mindful walking, noticing the sensation of your feet on the ground and the movement of your body. Even mundane tasks, such as washing dishes or brushing your teeth, can become opportunities for mindful awareness. By consciously focusing on the present moment during these activities, you gently shift your attention away from worries and anxieties, creating space for inner peace and calm.

Ayurveda encourages the integration of mindfulness and meditation into daily routines, particularly as part of the Dinacharya, the daily regimen. This might involve starting the day with a few minutes of meditation or incorporating mindful breathing throughout the day. Evening routines can also incorporate relaxation techniques such as a warm bath infused with calming herbs, followed by a short meditation session before bed. The consistency of these practices, even in small doses, helps to cultivate a sense of grounding and stability, buffering against the stresses of daily life.

It's important to note that Ayurveda doesn't prescribe a one-size-fits-all approach to mindfulness and meditation. The most effective practices are those that resonate with your individual constitution and preferences. Experiment with different techniques – guided meditations, mantra repetition, visualization, or body scans – to find what works best for you. Pay attention to how each practice makes you feel. If a particular technique increases your anxiety or restlessness, it may not be suitable for your dosha. Instead, explore alternative practices that promote a sense of calm and balance.

Furthermore, the benefits of mindfulness and meditation extend far beyond stress reduction. Regular practice can enhance self-awareness, improve focus and concentration, boost creativity, and foster emotional regulation. It can also contribute to better sleep, improved digestion, and enhanced overall well-being. These practices offer a profound and empowering way to cultivate inner resilience, enabling you to navigate the challenges of modern life with greater ease and grace. By integrating these practices into your life, you are not only managing stress but actively building a foundation for a healthier, more balanced, and fulfilling existence.

Consider integrating specific Ayurvedic techniques into your mindfulness and meditation practices. For example, incorporating the use of essential oils, such as lavender for Vata, sandalwood for Pitta, or rose for Kapha, can enhance the calming effects of your practice. Similarly, the use of specific mantras or visualizations, informed by your dosha, can deepen your connection to the present moment. For example, repeating a mantra associated with grounding and stability can be particularly helpful for Vata, while focusing on visualizations associated with coolness and calmness can be beneficial for Pitta. Kapha individuals may find visualizations of lightness and movement beneficial.

Remember, the journey towards mastering mindfulness and meditation is a gradual process. There will be days when you find it easier to focus, and other days when your mind wanders. Be patient and compassionate with yourself. Don't get discouraged if you struggle to maintain a still mind. The very act of noticing your mind wandering and gently redirecting your attention back to your breath or chosen focus is a practice in itself. This gentle redirection is the essence of mindfulness and will gradually strengthen your ability to focus and calm your mind over time. The consistency of your practice is what matters most. Even short, regular sessions are more effective than infrequent, lengthy ones.

Finally, remember to consult with a qualified Ayurvedic practitioner to personalize your stress management plan, including your mindfulness and meditation practices. They can guide you in choosing practices tailored to your unique dosha and constitution, and provide support and guidance as you embark on your journey towards a more balanced and peaceful life. The ancient wisdom of Ayurveda, coupled with the modern understanding of mindfulness and meditation, offers a powerful pathway to managing stress and cultivating a deeper sense of well-being. Embracing this holistic approach will not only reduce your stress levels but also pave the way for a more fulfilling and joyful life. The benefits will ripple outward, positively influencing every aspect of your health, relationships, and overall life experience.

The Role of Nature in Stress Relief

Ayurveda recognizes the profound connection between humans and nature, emphasizing the restorative power of the natural world in promoting balance and well-being. Chronic stress, a pervasive issue in modern life, disrupts this natural equilibrium, triggering a cascade of physiological and psychological imbalances. Fortunately, nature offers a wealth of resources to counteract these effects, providing a sanctuary for the stressed mind and body. Spending time outdoors is not merely a pleasant pastime; it's a vital component of an effective stress management strategy within the Ayurvedic framework.

The sensory experience of nature plays a crucial role in stress reduction. The sights, sounds, and smells of the natural world have a calming effect on the nervous system. The vibrant green hues of foliage, the gentle rustling of leaves, the melodious songs of birds, and the earthy aroma of soil all contribute to a sense of tranquility and peace. These sensory inputs activate the parasympathetic nervous system, counteracting the effects of the sympathetic nervous system, which is responsible for the body's stress response (fight-or-flight). Studies have shown that even brief exposure to nature can lower cortisol levels (the stress hormone) and reduce blood pressure, demonstrating the immediate physiological benefits of this connection.

Consider the impact of a walk in a forest. The phytoncides, aromatic volatile organic compounds released by trees, have been shown to have a positive effect on the immune system and reduce stress levels. This phenomenon, known as "forest bathing" or Shinrin-yoku, is increasingly recognized as a powerful tool for stress management and overall well-being.

The act of walking itself is beneficial, promoting physical activity and releasing endorphins, which have mood-boosting and pain-relieving effects. The uneven terrain, the gentle incline, and the variation in the walking surface stimulate different muscle groups, improving balance and coordination. This physical activity isn't solely for the body; it helps quiet a racing mind and encourages a meditative state, allowing one to feel more grounded and centered.

Beyond forests, other natural environments offer unique stress-reducing benefits. The rhythmic sound of ocean waves, the vast expanse of the sky, or the stillness of a mountain landscape all provide opportunities for reflection and relaxation. The vastness of nature often puts our worries into perspective, highlighting the insignificance of our daily stressors against the backdrop of the natural world. The calming effect of water, whether a flowing stream or a tranquil lake, is particularly potent. The sight and sound of water are deeply soothing, promoting a sense of peace and tranquility. The meditative quality of observing the gentle flow of a river or the lapping of waves on the shore can naturally quiet the mind, a practice in itself echoing the mindfulness techniques discussed earlier.

The choice of natural environment should be tailored to individual dosha constitutions. Vata individuals, characterized by their airy and restless nature, might find solace in the stillness of a mountain environment, or the grounding presence of a dense forest. The steady rhythm of the ocean waves could also help to calm their often scattered energy. Pitta individuals, known for their fiery and intense nature, might benefit from the cooling effect of water – a swim in a lake, a walk along a beach, or simply the sound of a gentle waterfall can provide a welcome sense of calm. Kapha individuals, who tend towards stability but can also become stagnant, may benefit from invigorating environments like hiking trails or brisk walks in sunny meadows, encouraging movement and uplifting their spirit.

Engaging all senses while in nature is crucial to maximize its therapeutic effect. Notice the textures of bark, leaves, and rocks under your feet. Listen carefully to the sounds of nature, from the gentle breeze to the distant calls of birds. Inhale deeply the scents of pine, earth, and flowers. Taste the fresh air, free from the pollutants of urban environments. Observe the intricate details of nature, appreciating the beauty and complexity of the natural world. This mindful interaction with nature transforms the experience from a passive observation into an active engagement, intensifying its healing effects.

Incorporating nature into daily routines is key to harnessing its stress-reducing power. Even small acts, like having a cup of tea on the balcony, taking a short walk during lunch, or simply sitting in a park to read a book, can make a significant difference. Gardening, a particularly therapeutic activity, offers a blend of physical activity and mindful engagement with nature. The act of planting seeds, nurturing plants, and harvesting fruits and vegetables fosters a sense of accomplishment and connection with the natural cycle of life. This connection further cultivates a sense of calm and purpose, reducing feelings of anxiety and stress.

Ayurveda recommends regular exposure to sunlight, which is crucial for Vitamin D synthesis and the regulation of the circadian rhythm. Sunlight helps regulate the body's internal clock, optimizing sleep-wake cycles and reducing stress associated with sleep disturbances. However, it's crucial to practice sun exposure safely, especially during peak hours. The Ayurvedic practice of spending time in the sun during specific times of the day, depending on the season and individual dosha, is a vital aspect of maintaining balance and well-being. Similarly, exposure to moonlight, particularly during the full moon, is considered beneficial, promoting emotional balance and reducing stress.

Beyond the sensory and physical benefits, spending time in nature offers a psychological sanctuary. It provides an opportunity to disconnect from the constant stimulation of technology and social media, fostering a sense of peace and solitude. The vastness of nature can put life's challenges into perspective, promoting feelings of gratitude and appreciation. This sense of perspective is invaluable in managing stress, as it allows us to see our worries with more clarity and objectivity, reducing their perceived impact on our well-being. It's an opportunity to reconnect with the simplicity and beauty of the world around us, reminding us of the inherent interconnectedness of all living things.

Furthermore, incorporating nature-inspired elements into our homes can also enhance our connection to the natural world, contributing to a sense of calmness and relaxation. The use of natural materials like wood, stone, and cotton in our decor, the incorporation of plants and flowers, and the use of natural light and ventilation all create a more harmonious and stress-reducing environment. These design choices are in line with Ayurvedic principles that emphasize living in harmony with nature. They help to create a space that feels soothing and restorative, promoting relaxation and stress reduction. Natural fragrances, such as essential oils derived from plants, can also be diffused to promote a sense of tranquility and well-being.

In conclusion, the role of nature in stress relief within the framework of Ayurveda is paramount. It's not merely a supplementary practice but an integral part of a holistic approach to well-being. By consciously incorporating time spent in nature into our daily routines, engaging our senses fully, and tailoring our experiences to our individual dosha constitutions, we can harness its profound stress-reducing and restorative properties. The natural world offers a sanctuary from the pressures of modern life, providing a pathway to greater balance, inner peace, and overall well-being. This approach is not only effective in reducing stress but also cultivates a deeper appreciation for the interconnectedness of life, enriching the entire human experience. The wisdom of Ayurveda lies in recognizing and utilizing this powerful connection to maintain equilibrium and find harmony amidst the chaos of daily life.

Herbal Remedies for Stress Management

Ayurveda offers a rich pharmacopoeia of herbs renowned for their ability to soothe the mind and calm the nervous system, effectively countering the detrimental effects of stress. These herbal remedies work on multiple levels, addressing both the physiological and psychological manifestations of stress. Understanding the individual dosha constitution is crucial in selecting the most appropriate herbal remedy, as the same herb may not be suitable for all individuals. A personalized approach, guided by an Ayurvedic practitioner, is highly recommended to ensure optimal efficacy and safety.

One of the most widely used herbs in Ayurvedic stress management is
Ashwagandha
(Withania somnifera). Known as "Indian ginseng," this adaptogen is celebrated for its ability to help the body adapt to stress. Ashwagandha
possesses potent anti-anxiety and anti-depressant properties, modulating the hypothalamic-pituitary-adrenal (HPA) axis—the body's central stress response system. Studies have demonstrated its effectiveness in reducing cortisol levels, the primary stress hormone, thereby promoting a sense of calm and well-being. Ashwagandha is particularly beneficial for individuals with Vata and Pitta doshas, who may experience heightened anxiety and irritability under stress. It is typically consumed as a powder, capsule, or in a herbal tea. However, it's crucial to consult a healthcare professional before using Ashwagandha, especially if pregnant, breastfeeding, or taking other medications. Individuals with autoimmune conditions should also exercise caution.

Another valuable herb is
Brahmi
(Bacopa monnieri), a powerful nervine tonic that enhances cognitive function and memory while simultaneously reducing stress and anxiety.

Brahmi promotes relaxation by gently calming the nervous system without causing drowsiness. It supports healthy brain function by improving neurotransmitter activity, bolstering memory and concentration, which can be significantly impaired under chronic stress. Brahmi is particularly effective for individuals with Vata dosha, who often experience mental agitation and scattered thoughts. It can be consumed as a powder, tablet, or liquid extract. While generally considered safe, it's advisable to consult an Ayurvedic practitioner before incorporating Brahmi into your routine, especially if you are taking medications that affect the central nervous system.

Jatamansi
(Nardostachys jatamansi) is a highly revered herb in Ayurveda, traditionally used to promote mental clarity, tranquility, and improved sleep quality. It is known for its calming and sedative effects, helping to alleviate anxiety and insomnia, often associated with chronic stress. Jatamansi is particularly useful for individuals with Vata and Pitta doshas, who may struggle with sleep disturbances and mental unrest.
It's commonly used in aromatherapy, as its fragrance is known for its calming properties. It can also be ingested as a powder or extract, always under the guidance of a qualified practitioner. While generally safe, it should be used cautiously by pregnant or breastfeeding women and those with specific medical conditions.

Tulsi
(Ocimum tenuiflorum), or holy basil, is a sacred herb in Ayurvedic tradition, revered for its ability to adapt to stress and boost immunity. It possesses potent antioxidant and anti-inflammatory properties, helping to counteract the physiological damage caused by chronic stress. Tulsi helps balance the doshas and is particularly beneficial for individuals with Vata and Pitta, offering relief from anxiety and improving respiratory function, often compromised during stress. It can be consumed as a tea, adding a few fresh

leaves to hot water or using commercially available Tulsi tea bags. The leaves can also be added to food. Tulsi is generally safe for consumption, but individuals with certain medical conditions should consult with a healthcare professional before regular use.

Gotu Kola
(Centella asiatica) is another remarkable herb that enhances cognitive function and supports the nervous system's health. It is traditionally used to improve memory, concentration, and mental clarity, all of which can be significantly affected by chronic stress. Gotu Kola promotes relaxation and has a gentle uplifting effect on mood, reducing anxiety and irritability. It's particularly beneficial for individuals with Vata and Kapha doshas. It's commonly consumed as a capsule or liquid extract, often combined with other stress-reducing herbs. While generally safe, pregnant and breastfeeding women should exercise caution and consult with a healthcare practitioner before use.

The appropriate use of these herbs should always be under the guidance of a qualified Ayurvedic practitioner. Self-medication can be risky, and the correct dosage and combination of herbs depend on the individual's dosha, constitution, and specific health concerns. An Ayurvedic practitioner will consider the individual's unique needs and circumstances to create a personalized herbal regimen that complements other stress management techniques such as yoga, meditation, and lifestyle adjustments.

Furthermore, the preparation and consumption methods are vital for maximizing the therapeutic benefits of these herbs. For instance, certain herbs may be more effective when consumed in the morning, while others may be more suitable for evening use. The practitioner will also advise on the ideal form of the herb—powder, capsule, tea, or extract—based on individual needs and preferences.

The effectiveness of these herbal remedies can be significantly enhanced by integrating them into a holistic Ayurvedic lifestyle. A balanced diet, regular exercise tailored to one's dosha, sufficient sleep, and mindfulness practices play a crucial role in creating a resilient mind and body capable of better managing stress. This integrated approach supports the body's natural ability to cope with stress, maximizing the benefits of the herbal remedies.

Beyond the specific herbs mentioned, numerous other plants and botanicals are used in Ayurveda to support stress management. For example, Valerian root is sometimes recommended for its sleep-promoting properties, while Lavender and Chamomile are commonly used in aromatherapy for their calming effects. However, it's crucial to remember that these herbs may interact with other medications and underlying health conditions. It is imperative to consult with an Ayurvedic practitioner before utilizing any herbal remedy for stress relief.

Ayurveda emphasizes a personalized approach, recognizing that each individual responds differently to herbal therapies. What works well for one person may not be as effective for another. Therefore, a thorough assessment by a qualified practitioner is essential to determine the most appropriate herbal remedies and dosage for each individual. This individualized approach ensures the safe and effective management of stress and the promotion of holistic well-being.

The integration of herbal remedies into a broader Ayurvedic lifestyle significantly enhances their effectiveness. A holistic approach, incorporating diet, exercise, sleep hygiene, and stress-reduction techniques, creates a supportive environment for the herbs to work optimally. The herbs themselves then become a powerful tool within a comprehensive strategy for managing stress effectively and sustainably. This comprehensive strategy, guided by the principles of Ayurveda, empowers individuals to navigate the challenges of modern life with greater resilience and inner peace. The understanding and application of these principles pave the way for a more harmonious relationship with oneself and the natural world, leading to a more balanced and fulfilling life. Ayurveda provides a roadmap for reclaiming control over one's health and well-being, empowering individuals to take an active role in creating a life characterized by tranquility and vitality. This empowerment is a cornerstone of the Ayurvedic philosophy, recognizing the innate capacity within each individual to achieve optimal health.

This personalized approach underscores the wisdom of Ayurveda, offering a gentle yet profound way to alleviate the pervasive problem of stress. By carefully considering individual needs and combining herbal remedies with a supportive lifestyle, individuals can effectively manage stress, reducing its damaging impact on both physical and mental health. The integration of Ayurveda's time-tested methods into modern life provides a holistic, effective, and sustainable path to greater well-being, reinforcing the harmony between mind, body, and spirit. This harmonious integration is the essence of Ayurvedic healing, allowing individuals to live in greater balance and vitality amidst the often-chaotic demands of daily life. The pursuit of this balance is not merely a goal; it is a journey, guided by the ancient wisdom of Ayurveda and informed by the individual's unique needs and aspirations.

Creating a Personalized Stress Management Plan

Building upon the foundation of understanding your dosha and incorporating appropriate herbal remedies, the next crucial step in managing stress within the Ayurvedic framework is crafting a personalized stress management plan. This isn't a one-size-fits-all approach; rather, it's a deeply individualistic process that requires introspection, self-awareness, and a willingness to experiment to discover what truly works for you. Remember, the goal isn't to eliminate stress entirely—that's unrealistic and arguably unhealthy—but to develop resilience and coping mechanisms that allow you to navigate stressful situations with grace and balance.

The creation of your personalized plan begins with honest self-assessment. Consider your daily routine, identifying triggers that consistently elevate your stress levels. Are these triggers related to work, relationships, financial pressures, or health concerns? Keeping a journal for a week or two, meticulously noting your daily activities, emotional states, and the situations that induce stress, can provide invaluable insights. Pay close attention to the time of day when stress tends to peak, and the specific physical and emotional sensations associated with it. Do you experience headaches, muscle tension, digestive upset, or a racing heart? Is your stress accompanied by irritability, anxiety, or feelings of overwhelm? These details are crucial for understanding your individual response to stress.

Once you have a clear picture of your stress triggers and responses, you can start to build a tailored plan. This plan should encompass several key areas: lifestyle adjustments, dietary modifications, herbal remedies (as discussed previously), and stress-reducing practices.

Let's delve into lifestyle adjustments. The Ayurvedic concept of *Dinacharya*, or daily routine, plays a pivotal role in stress management. A consistent and mindful daily routine helps regulate your circadian rhythm, promoting hormonal balance and reducing cortisol levels, the primary stress hormone.

This routine should include a regular sleep schedule—aiming for 7-8 hours of uninterrupted sleep—with a consistent bedtime and wake-up time, even on weekends. Incorporate regular physical activity suited to your dosha. Vata types might benefit from gentle yoga or walking, while Pitta types might find relief in swimming or cycling. Kapha types could engage in more vigorous activities like running or team sports. Remember, the key is consistency and finding an activity that you enjoy.

Dietary modifications are equally crucial. Ayurveda emphasizes the importance of a balanced diet consisting of all six tastes: sweet, sour, salty, pungent, bitter, and astringent. A diet lacking in any of these tastes can contribute to imbalances and exacerbate stress. Prioritize whole, unprocessed foods that are seasonal and locally sourced. Reduce your intake of processed foods, refined sugars, caffeine, and alcohol, all of which can significantly impact your stress levels and disrupt your hormonal balance. Incorporating foods known for their calming properties, such as milk (especially warm milk with turmeric or cardamom), ghee (clarified butter), and sweet potatoes, can be highly beneficial. Spices like coriander, cumin, and fennel are also known for their digestive and calming effects. For Vata types, focus on warming, grounding foods; for Pitta, cooling and soothing foods; and for Kapha, foods that are light and easily digestible.

Your personalized stress management plan should also integrate the herbal remedies discussed in the previous chapter. However, remember the critical role of individualization. What works for one person might not work for another. If you're unsure about which herbs are suitable for your dosha and specific needs, consulting a qualified Ayurvedic practitioner is essential. They can assess your unique constitution and recommend appropriate herbs in safe and effective dosages. Never self-prescribe herbal remedies, especially if you are taking other medications.

Beyond lifestyle changes and dietary modifications, the inclusion of stress-reducing practices is vital. These practices are designed to calm the nervous system and promote a sense of inner peace. Consider incorporating practices like yoga, pranayama (breathing exercises), meditation, or spending time in nature. Yoga, particularly restorative yoga, can help release muscle tension and calm the mind. Pranayama techniques, such as alternate nostril breathing (Nadi Shodhana), can balance the energy flow in the body and reduce anxiety. Meditation, even for just a few minutes a day, can help quiet the mind and cultivate a sense of presence. Spending time in nature, whether it's a walk in the park or sitting by a quiet body of water, has been shown to reduce stress hormones and promote relaxation.

The creation of a personalized stress management plan is an ongoing process, not a one-time event. Regularly reassess your plan and make adjustments as needed. What works well at one point in your life may not be as effective later on. Pay attention to your body's signals and adapt your plan accordingly. Keep a journal to track your progress and note any changes in your stress levels. Remember that consistency is key. The more consistently you implement the various components of your plan, the greater the benefits you will experience.

It's also important to build in self-compassion. Don't get discouraged if you have setbacks. Life is inherently unpredictable, and there will be times when stress levels rise despite your best efforts. The key is to treat these setbacks as opportunities for learning and growth. Rather than beating yourself up, acknowledge the situation, adjust your plan if necessary, and gently guide yourself back to balance.

For those with particularly high stress levels or chronic stress-related conditions, seeking professional help is crucial. An Ayurvedic practitioner can provide personalized guidance and support, ensuring your plan is tailored to your unique needs. They can also help identify underlying imbalances that may be contributing to your stress. In addition to Ayurvedic interventions, consider consulting with other healthcare professionals, such as a therapist or counselor, to address the psychological and emotional aspects of stress. A holistic approach, integrating Ayurvedic principles with other forms of therapy, can provide the most comprehensive and effective stress management strategy.

To illustrate the creation of a personalized plan, let's consider three individuals with different dosha constitutions and stress responses:

Individual 1: Predominantly Vata Dosha

This individual experiences stress as anxiety, nervousness, and insomnia. They might find themselves feeling scattered and overwhelmed, with racing thoughts and difficulty concentrating. Their stress triggers might include deadlines, travel, or unpredictable events.

Their personalized plan might include:

Lifestyle:
A consistent bedtime routine, incorporating warm milk with ashwagandha before bed, gentle yoga practices like restorative yoga or Yin yoga, and prioritizing a calm and organized environment.

Diet:
Emphasis on warming, grounding foods like soups, stews, and cooked vegetables. Inclusion of foods rich in healthy fats like avocados and nuts. Limiting caffeine and alcohol intake.

Herbs:
Ashwagandha, Shatavari, and Brahmi are commonly used to calm Vata dosha. Always consult a qualified practitioner before using these herbs.

Stress-reducing practices:
Meditation, deep breathing exercises, and spending time in nature.

Individual 2: Predominantly Pitta Dosha

This individual might experience stress as anger, irritability, and frustration. Their stress triggers could include conflict, intense competition, or excessive heat. They might exhibit physical symptoms such as heartburn, skin rashes, or headaches.

Their personalized plan could include:

Lifestyle:
Prioritizing a cool and calm environment, avoiding overstimulation, and incorporating regular breaks throughout the day. Engaging in activities that promote relaxation and self-care, such as spending time in nature.

Diet:
Focus on cooling foods like fruits, vegetables, and dairy products. Minimizing spicy and pungent foods. Staying well-hydrated.

Herbs:
Amalaki, Guggul, and Brahmi can be beneficial for calming Pitta. Again, consulting a practitioner is crucial.

Stress-reducing practices:
Swimming, gentle yoga, meditation, and spending time in cool, tranquil
environments.

Individual 3: Predominantly Kapha Dosha

This individual might experience stress as lethargy, sluggishness, and difficulty concentrating. Their stress triggers could include monotony, inactivity, or feeling overwhelmed by routine. They might struggle with feelings of sadness or depression.

Their plan might include:

Lifestyle:
Prioritizing activities that stimulate their energy levels. Regular exercise, particularly vigorous forms of exercise. Maintaining a clean and organized environment. **Diet:**
Emphasis on light, easily digestible foods. Reducing intake of heavy, greasy foods, and dairy products.
Herbs:
Ginger, Turmeric, and Arjuna can be helpful for stimulating Kapha. Seek professional guidance for appropriate use.
Stress-reducing practices:
Fast-paced yoga styles, brisk walks, and invigorating activities.

Remember, these are just examples. Your personalized stress management plan should be uniquely tailored to your individual needs, preferences, and dosha constitution. The journey towards stress management is a journey of self-discovery, a continuous process of refinement and adaptation. By understanding your body's unique signals and working closely with a qualified practitioner if needed, you can cultivate resilience and navigate the challenges of daily life with greater ease and inner harmony. The ultimate goal is not the eradication of stress but the development of a balanced state of being, one where you feel empowered to meet life's challenges with equanimity and grace, allowing you to flourish within the chaotic world around you.

The Ayurvedic Cleansing Process

Panchakarma, often translated as "five actions," is the cornerstone of Ayurvedic detoxification. It's not merely a cleanse; it's a deeply transformative process designed to restore balance within the body, mind, and spirit. This ancient system of therapies aims to remove accumulated toxins (ama) from the tissues, revitalize the body's natural healing mechanisms, and promote overall well-being. Think of it not as a quick fix, but as a profound journey towards restoring your inherent equilibrium. The process is deeply personalized, tailored to the individual's unique constitution (dosha) and current state of health. There's no one-size-fits-all approach to Panchakarma; a skilled Ayurvedic practitioner will carefully assess your needs before recommending a specific course of treatment.

The philosophy behind Panchakarma is rooted in the Ayurvedic understanding of the body's intricate interconnectedness. It recognizes that imbalances in one area can ripple through the entire system, leading to a cascade of health issues. By systematically eliminating accumulated toxins, Panchakarma creates space for the body to heal itself and regain its inherent balance. This holistic approach considers not only the physical body but also the mental and emotional aspects of well-being. The process often includes dietary adjustments, lifestyle modifications, and herbal remedies in conjunction with the therapeutic procedures.

The five main therapies that form the core of Panchakarma are Vamana (therapeutic emesis), Virechana (therapeutic purgation), Basti (therapeutic enema), Nasya (nasal administration), and Raktamokshana (bloodletting). Each therapy targets specific channels and tissues within the body, working to eliminate toxins and restore flow. These therapies are not always necessary or suitable for everyone; the practitioner will determine which, if any, are appropriate based on individual needs. Let's delve a little deeper into each of these five primary therapies:

Vamana, or therapeutic emesis, involves inducing vomiting to eliminate excess Kapha dosha and toxins accumulated in the upper body. It's primarily indicated for conditions involving excess mucus, such as respiratory ailments, allergies, and certain skin conditions. Vamana isn't a haphazard process; it's carefully managed by a skilled practitioner using specific herbal preparations to promote a gentle and effective clearing of the upper respiratory tract. This isn't about inducing vomiting at will; it's a precise, medically guided procedure designed to achieve specific therapeutic outcomes. This therapy is often accompanied by a specific diet and lifestyle changes both before and after the procedure.

Virechana, or therapeutic purgation, focuses on eliminating toxins accumulated in the lower gastrointestinal tract. This therapy involves the administration of herbal purgatives to induce bowel movements, promoting the elimination of excess Pitta dosha and toxins from the lower body. Like Vamana, Virechana is carefully planned and supervised by a qualified practitioner. The goal isn't simply to induce diarrhea; it's a controlled process that aims to cleanse the digestive tract effectively and gently. The practitioner will work with you to determine the appropriate herbal preparation and dosage based on your constitution and health condition. Pre and post-treatment dietary guidelines are vital components of the success of this therapy.

Basti, or therapeutic enema, is a powerful therapy that targets the colon. It involves the administration of medicated enemas to cleanse the large intestine and balance Vata dosha. Basti is often used to treat chronic constipation, inflammatory bowel disorders, and various other conditions affecting the lower gastrointestinal tract. The medicated enemas are carefully formulated with herbs that have specific therapeutic properties, designed to soothe and cleanse the colon while promoting optimal functioning. The type and formulation of the enema are carefully chosen based on the individual's needs and dosha. The process is typically administered over a course of several days, promoting gradual and thorough cleansing.

Nasya, or nasal administration, is a therapy that involves instilling medicated oils or herbal preparations into the nasal passages. This therapy is aimed at balancing Vata and Kapha doshas, relieving congestion in the head and neck, and improving overall clarity and mental function. The medicated oils used in Nasya are carefully selected to address specific imbalances and ailments. Regular practice of Nasya is believed to promote sensory acuity, reduce headaches, and improve cognitive function. This is often considered a preventative therapy, beneficial for overall health and well-being. This gentle yet powerful therapy offers a multitude of benefits, promoting both physical and mental clarity.

Raktamokshana, or bloodletting, is a more advanced Panchakarma therapy that involves removing small amounts of blood from the body. It's not a common therapy and is only used in specific circumstances and under the strict supervision of a highly qualified Ayurvedic practitioner. This therapy is used cautiously and only when absolutely necessary for conditions involving excess Pitta or when toxins are deeply entrenched in the blood. The process is precisely controlled to avoid any adverse effects. The practitioner will assess the individual's health thoroughly before recommending this therapy. It's important to understand that this is a specialized treatment and not a generally recommended part of Panchakarma for the average individual.

Preparation for Panchakarma is crucial for its success. This preparation phase, often referred to as Purva Karma, involves dietary adjustments, lifestyle changes, and sometimes herbal remedies designed to prepare the body for the detoxification process. The aim is to gently shift the body into a state where it is better able to release toxins. This phase may involve increased consumption of warm water, lighter meals, and gentle exercise. Specific dietary recommendations will depend on your dosha and the chosen therapy. For example, individuals may be advised to reduce the intake of certain foods that could interfere with the detoxification process. This period of preparation is equally important as the therapy itself, allowing for a smooth and effective experience.

Post-Panchakarma care, or Paschat Karma, is just as vital as the therapy itself. It's a period of careful nurturing to help the body integrate the benefits of the treatment and prevent the accumulation of toxins again. This phase often includes a specific diet, herbal supplements, and lifestyle modifications to support the body's natural healing processes. The dietary recommendations during this phase usually focus on easily digestible foods that support the body's ability to assimilate nutrients and eliminate waste products. Gentle exercise, sufficient rest, and stress-reducing practices are also encouraged. A skilled practitioner will provide personalized guidance to ensure a smooth transition back to a healthy and balanced lifestyle.

Finding a qualified Ayurvedic practitioner is paramount when considering Panchakarma. This is not a self-treatment;

the therapies should be administered by experienced professionals who understand the nuances of this complex system. A qualified practitioner will conduct a thorough assessment of your health, considering your dosha, current health conditions, and lifestyle to recommend the appropriate therapies and develop a personalized treatment plan. Their guidance is essential for ensuring safety, efficacy, and achieving optimal results. Don't hesitate to ask questions and discuss any concerns you may have before proceeding with any Panchakarma treatment.

In conclusion, Panchakarma is a powerful and profound system of Ayurvedic detoxification that can significantly impact overall health and well-being. It's a deeply personalized process that should be approached with respect and guidance from a qualified practitioner. By combining specific therapies with dietary adjustments and lifestyle changes, Panchakarma aims not only to remove toxins but to restore balance, promote healing, and enhance vitality. The transformative potential of this ancient system makes it a truly valuable tool for those seeking a deeper level of health and wellness. Remember, this is a journey, not a race; a well-planned and carefully executed Panchakarma process can lead to remarkable improvements in health, energy levels, and overall quality of life.

The Five Main Panchakarma Therapies

The effectiveness of Panchakarma hinges on its precise application, tailored to the individual's unique constitution and health condition. A qualified Ayurvedic practitioner plays a crucial role in this process, conducting a thorough assessment to determine the appropriate therapies and their sequence. This personalized approach ensures optimal results and minimizes any potential discomfort. Let's delve into the five primary Panchakarma therapies: Vamana (therapeutic emesis), Virechana (therapeutic purgation), Basti (medicated enemas), Nasya (nasal administration), and Raktamokshana (bloodletting).

Vamana, or therapeutic emesis, is indicated for Kapha and Kapha-Pitta imbalances characterized by excessive mucus accumulation in the respiratory tract, digestive system, and skin. It involves inducing vomiting through the careful administration of herbal emetics. This therapy is not a forceful expulsion but a gentle and controlled process, aimed at eliminating excess Kapha dosha and associated toxins. It's crucial to understand that Vamana is not a method for weight loss; its primary purpose is to cleanse the body of accumulated Kapha dosha. The process typically involves a preparatory phase of dietary adjustments and herbal preparations to prepare the body for the emesis procedure itself. This preparatory phase is critical for maximizing the effectiveness and minimizing potential discomfort. Following Vamana, a carefully planned post-treatment diet is essential to support the body's rebalancing process. This often involves easily digestible foods, and avoidance of heavy or mucus-forming substances. Individuals with conditions like heart disease, ulcers, or severe dehydration are generally not candidates for Vamana.

Virechana, therapeutic purgation, targets Pitta dosha imbalances and is particularly beneficial for conditions characterized by excessive heat and inflammation. This therapy involves the administration of herbal purgatives to induce bowel movements, eliminating toxins accumulated in the gastrointestinal tract. Like Vamana, Virechana is a controlled and carefully guided process, not a harsh or indiscriminate purging. The practitioner will select specific herbal formulations tailored to the individual's unique constitution and the nature of their imbalance. The preparatory phase for Virechana involves a specific diet, designed to prepare the digestive system for the procedure and enhance its effectiveness. The post-treatment phase emphasizes rehydration and a diet that supports the digestive system's healing and rebalancing process. Individuals with conditions such as dehydration, inflammatory bowel disease, or severe diarrhea are generally not suitable candidates for Virechana.

Basti, medicated enemas, is a crucial therapy in Panchakarma, particularly beneficial for Vata dosha imbalances and conditions affecting the lower abdomen and colon. It involves the administration of medicated liquids into the rectum, which helps to cleanse the colon and restore proper bowel function. The herbal preparations used in Basti vary depending on the specific condition and the individual's dosha. Some formulations are designed to soothe and lubricate the colon, while others address specific imbalances or conditions like constipation, irritable bowel syndrome, or inflammation. Basti is often administered as a series of treatments, allowing for a deeper and more comprehensive cleansing effect. A thorough assessment by an Ayurvedic practitioner is crucial to determine the appropriate type of Basti and the duration of the treatment. Contraindications for

Basti might include certain bowel conditions such as severe colitis or recent abdominal surgery.

Nasya, nasal administration, focuses on the head and upper respiratory tract, addressing Vata and Kapha imbalances that manifest as headaches, sinus congestion, and neurological disorders. It involves the administration of medicated oils or herbal preparations through the nostrils. The oils used in Nasya often contain herbs with specific properties, such as anti-inflammatory, analgesic, or nervine effects. This therapy is known to enhance sensory perception, improve circulation to the head and neck, and promote mental clarity. Nasya is a gentle and well-tolerated procedure when administered by a qualified practitioner. However, certain conditions such as severe nosebleeds or acute sinusitis may preclude the use of this therapy. The post-treatment care usually involves avoiding cold exposure and maintaining a balanced diet.

Raktamokshana, or bloodletting, is a more advanced and less frequently employed Panchakarma therapy. It's used selectively to address certain specific conditions and requires meticulous skill and judgment from the Ayurvedic practitioner. This therapy involves removing small amounts of blood from the body, generally to balance Pitta dosha and reduce excessive heat and inflammation. It's not a generalized blood-letting practice but targeted towards specific conditions and following a careful evaluation by the practitioner. The practitioner assesses the individual's blood constitution and determines the necessity and the appropriate amount of blood to be removed. It's important to note that Raktamokshana is only performed under strict conditions and by highly skilled practitioners. This therapy is generally avoided in individuals with anemia or other blood-related disorders.

The success of Panchakarma depends not only on the therapies themselves but also on the preparation and post-treatment phases. The preparatory phase involves a specific diet and lifestyle adjustments to prepare the body for the treatments. This usually includes a period of cleansing, with emphasis on easily digestible foods, avoidance of stimulants, and sufficient rest. After the Panchakarma therapies, a transitional diet and lifestyle are essential to support the body's rebalancing process and maintain the positive effects of the detoxification. This typically includes gentle exercise, stress management techniques, and a continued emphasis on nourishing foods that support the individual's constitution. The duration of the preparatory and post-treatment phases depends on the individual's condition and the specific therapies used. A qualified Ayurvedic practitioner will create a tailored plan based on the individual's needs.

It's crucial to emphasize the importance of seeking guidance from a qualified and experienced Ayurvedic practitioner before undertaking any Panchakarma therapies. These therapies are potent and should only be performed under proper supervision to ensure safety and maximize benefits. The practitioner will assess the individual's health history, current condition, and doshic constitution, determining the appropriate therapies, their sequence, and the duration of the treatment. They will also guide the individual through the preparatory and post-treatment phases, ensuring optimal results and minimizing potential discomfort or complications. A proper understanding of the process and working with a trained professional ensures that the experience is a transformative one, leading to improved overall health, energy levels, and a deeper sense of well-being. The transformative power of Panchakarma lies in its holistic approach, addressing not only physical imbalances but also mental and emotional aspects. The goal is to restore the body's inherent capacity for self-healing and establish a foundation for lasting wellness. The integration of Panchakarma with lifestyle modifications and dietary changes ensures long-term benefits, supporting overall vitality and resilience. The journey to better health through Ayurveda involves a commitment to personalized care, meticulous planning, and a close working relationship with a skilled practitioner.

Dietary and Lifestyle Guidelines

Preparing for Panchakarma is a crucial step in ensuring the effectiveness and safety of this powerful Ayurvedic detoxification process. It's not merely about undergoing the therapies themselves; it's about preparing the body and mind to fully receive their benefits. This preparation involves a period of dietary and lifestyle adjustments designed to cleanse and balance the doshas, creating an optimal environment for the therapies to work their magic. This preparatory phase, often lasting several days or even weeks depending on the individual's condition and the chosen Panchakarma therapies, is as important as the therapies themselves. Think of it as meticulously preparing the soil before planting a seed – ensuring the best possible conditions for growth and flourishing.

The dietary adjustments during the preparatory phase are tailored to the individual's unique doshic constitution and current state of health. However, certain general principles apply across the board. The emphasis shifts towards easily digestible foods that are light, warm, and nourishing. This ensures that the digestive system is not overburdened during the detoxification process, allowing the body to focus its energy on elimination rather than digestion. Heavy, greasy, fried, processed, and overly spicy foods are typically avoided. These foods can create ama (toxins) that hinder the effectiveness of the Panchakarma therapies.

Specific dietary recommendations vary depending on the dosha. For instance, individuals with a predominantly Vata constitution, characterized by dryness and movement, might benefit from warm, cooked foods with grounding qualities, such as soups, stews, and well-cooked grains like quinoa or brown rice. Pitta individuals, known for their fiery nature, might find solace in cooling foods like cucumbers, spinach, and coconut water. Kapha individuals, often characterized by heaviness and sluggishness, benefit from lighter, warming foods that help stimulate their digestive fire, such as ginger, turmeric, and spices in moderation.

The importance of consuming fresh, seasonal fruits and vegetables cannot be overstated. These foods are rich in vitamins, minerals, and antioxidants that support the body's natural detoxification processes. Freshly squeezed juices, particularly those made from fruits and vegetables appropriate for the individual's dosha, can also be incorporated into the diet. However, it's essential to avoid excessive consumption of fruits, particularly those with high sugar content, which could potentially increase ama production.

Hydration is another critical aspect of Panchakarma preparation. Drinking plenty of warm water throughout the day is essential for flushing out toxins and supporting the elimination process. Herbal teas, especially those with digestive and detoxifying properties like ginger, chamomile, or fennel, can be beneficial. Avoiding cold drinks and iced beverages is crucial as they can suppress the digestive fire (Agni). The focus is always on maintaining a balanced and harmonious internal environment, nurturing the body's natural cleansing capabilities.

Beyond diet, lifestyle adjustments play a crucial role in optimizing the Panchakarma experience. Reducing stress is paramount. Stress weakens the digestive system and hinders the body's ability to eliminate toxins effectively. Incorporating stress-reduction techniques such as meditation, yoga, deep breathing exercises, or spending time in nature can greatly enhance the efficacy of Panchakarma. Regular gentle exercise is also encouraged, but strenuous activities should be avoided, particularly as the Panchakarma therapies approach. The goal is to gently support the body's natural cleansing processes without overexerting it.

Sleep is a vital aspect of the preparatory phase. Aiming for at least seven to eight hours of quality sleep each night is essential for allowing the body to rest, repair, and rejuvenate. A consistent sleep schedule and a relaxing bedtime routine can significantly contribute to improved sleep quality. Creating a serene and calming bedroom environment, free from electronic devices and bright lights, is advisable. Adequate sleep is not merely a luxurious addition; it is an integral part of the healing process, promoting overall well-being and supporting the body's natural detoxification mechanisms.

The preparatory phase also involves paying close attention to the routines of daily life. This encompasses aspects of Dinacharya, the daily Ayurvedic regimen. Maintaining a regular routine, including consistent wake up and bedtime times, promotes balance and harmony within the body. Regular oil massage (Abhyanga) can be beneficial, as it helps to lubricate the tissues and promote the elimination of toxins through the skin. Gentle self-massage can be a soothing and grounding practice, particularly during the preparatory phase. The emphasis on consistency in daily activities helps establish an equilibrium, setting the stage for the Panchakarma therapies to be most effective.

In the weeks leading up to Panchakarma, it is advisable to gradually reduce the consumption of stimulants such as caffeine and alcohol. These substances can disrupt the digestive system and hinder the body's ability to detoxify. Furthermore, it's beneficial to reduce exposure to environmental toxins, including pollutants in the air and harmful chemicals in personal care products. Minimizing exposure to these toxins allows the body to focus its energy on the internal detoxification process, promoting a more effective and thorough cleanse.

One of the essential preparations is mental and emotional readiness. Panchakarma can be a transformative experience, both physically and emotionally. During the therapies, emotional issues can sometimes surface as the body releases accumulated toxins. This is often a sign of progress and a testament to the therapies' deep cleansing effect. It is advisable to incorporate practices that promote emotional well-being, such as meditation, mindfulness exercises, or journaling. Taking time to reflect on one's emotional state and to address any underlying stressors can make a significant difference in the overall experience.

Furthermore, during the preparatory phase, it's important to connect with the practitioner overseeing the Panchakarma therapies. Regular communication, ideally in-person consultations, enables the practitioner to monitor the individual's progress and make any necessary adjustments to the preparation plan. This collaborative approach emphasizes the importance of a personalized journey, tailored to the unique needs and responses of the individual. The practitioner can provide guidance, answer questions, and offer support, enhancing the overall effectiveness and comfort of the experience.

The preparatory phase should not be viewed as a restrictive period of deprivation, but rather as a period of nurturing and preparation. It's an opportunity to consciously choose foods and activities that support the body's natural cleansing and rejuvenation processes. By diligently following the dietary and lifestyle guidelines, individuals can significantly enhance the effectiveness of the Panchakarma therapies, maximizing their potential benefits for achieving lasting health and well-being. The transformative potential of Panchakarma lies not just in the therapies themselves, but also in the mindful preparation that precedes them, setting the stage for a deeply restorative and healing experience. The process, while demanding at times, ultimately serves as a testament to the power of self-care and the body's innate capacity for healing. This preparatory phase is an integral part of the entire Panchakarma process; therefore, meticulous attention to detail is crucial for a successful and transformative outcome. The dedication shown during this phase reflects the commitment to holistic well-being and establishes a foundation for long-term health and vitality.

Maintaining the Benefits

The completion of your Panchakarma therapies marks not an end, but a beginning – the beginning of a sustained journey towards enhanced well-being. The transformative effects of this deep detoxification process are best preserved through a carefully considered post-treatment care plan. This phase is as critical as the therapies themselves, acting as a bridge to integrate the benefits achieved and prevent a relapse into old patterns. Think of it as nurturing a delicate seedling after transplanting – gentle care ensures its growth into a strong, healthy plant.

The immediate post-Panchakarma period is characterized by a heightened sensitivity. Your body, having undergone a profound cleansing, is more receptive to both positive and negative influences. This is why meticulous adherence to recommended guidelines is paramount. The goal is to support the body's natural healing mechanisms, allowing it to fully integrate the benefits of the therapies. This includes gentle reintroduction of foods, gradual resumption of activities, and a continued emphasis on stress reduction and mindful living.

Dietary recommendations during this phase focus on easily digestible foods that are nourishing and gentle on the digestive system. Avoid anything heavy, greasy, or overly stimulating. Think light soups, well-cooked vegetables, kitchari (a simple mung bean and rice porridge), and easily digestible grains like rice and oats. These foods minimize the workload on the digestive system, allowing it to focus on healing and rebalancing. Spices like ginger, cardamom, and cumin can be incorporated to enhance digestion and promote a sense of warmth and wellbeing. These spices aid in the assimilation of nutrients and support the body's natural detoxification pathways.

Avoid all processed foods, refined sugars, caffeine, alcohol, and red meat. These substances are known to place stress on the digestive system and may impede the healing process. Focus on fresh, seasonal produce, choosing foods that are appropriate for your dominant dosha. For example, if you are predominantly Vata, warm, cooked foods are preferable, whereas Pitta may benefit from cooling foods like cucumber and coconut water. Kapha types may find lighter, more warming foods to be beneficial. This is a time to listen to your body and adjust your diet accordingly, taking note of how different foods make you feel.

The transition back to a regular diet should be gradual. Begin by adding a new food each day, observing its effect on your digestion and overall well-being. If you experience any discomfort, such as bloating, gas, or indigestion, it's a sign to slow down and stick with easily digestible options for a longer period. Remember, patience and gentle self-care are key elements in the post-Panchakarma recovery process. Rushing back into old habits can easily undo the benefits of the therapies.

Beyond dietary modifications, lifestyle adjustments are equally important for sustaining the effects of Panchakarma. Adequate sleep is crucial for allowing the body to rest and repair. Aim for 7-8 hours of quality sleep each night, establishing a regular sleep schedule to regulate your circadian rhythm. Engage in gentle exercise, such as yoga or walking, to promote circulation and lymphatic drainage. Avoid strenuous exercise that could overtax the system. Remember, the goal is to gently support the body's healing processes, not to push it beyond its limits.

Stress management is another key element of post-Panchakarma care. Ayurveda recognizes the profound connection between stress and imbalance. Chronic stress can disrupt the delicate equilibrium achieved through Panchakarma, undoing much of the therapeutic benefits. Incorporate stress-reducing practices into your daily routine. This could include meditation, deep breathing exercises, spending time in nature, or engaging in activities you find relaxing and enjoyable.

Remember the importance of Abhyanga, the Ayurvedic self-massage. Gentle self-massage with warm, sesame oil can continue to promote circulation and relaxation. This daily practice further supports the body's natural healing processes. It also aids in nourishing the skin and promoting a sense of overall well-being. The oil used should be tailored to your dosha, ensuring a gentle and calming effect.

Hydration is also paramount. Drink plenty of warm water throughout the day to support detoxification and overall health. Warm water helps to flush out toxins and aids in digestion. Herbal teas, such as ginger tea or chamomile tea, can also be beneficial. Avoid cold beverages which can dampen the digestive fire.

The post-Panchakarma period is an ideal time to focus on establishing healthy daily routines, known as Dinacharya. This involves creating a structured daily schedule that incorporates activities that support balance and well-being. This includes regular waking and sleeping times, mindful eating, daily exercise, and stress-reducing practices. The consistency of these routines helps to solidify the positive changes achieved through Panchakarma, preventing a return to old, unhealthy habits.

Consider incorporating additional Ayurvedic practices into your daily routine, such as Nasya (nasal administration of medicated oils), which can help to clear the sinuses and improve respiratory health. Similarly, Shirodhara (a continuous stream of warm oil poured onto the forehead) can be extremely helpful for relaxation and stress reduction. However, these should be undertaken under the guidance of a qualified Ayurvedic practitioner.

Maintaining a positive mental attitude is also crucial. Panchakarma is a transformative journey, and a positive mindset can significantly enhance its long-term benefits. Engage in activities that bring you joy, practice gratitude, and connect with loved ones. Surround yourself with a supportive community that understands and appreciates your commitment to holistic well-being.

Finally, consider keeping a journal to track your progress and identify any potential challenges. This allows you to observe patterns in your energy levels, digestion, and overall sense of well-being. This valuable information aids in making necessary adjustments to your diet and lifestyle as needed. It also allows you to appreciate the transformative journey you've undertaken and serves as a testament to your commitment to your own health and well-being.

The post-Panchakarma phase is not a quick fix, but a gradual integration of healthy habits and a mindful approach to life. By diligently following these recommendations, you can solidify the transformative effects of Panchakarma, leading to a life of increased vitality, improved well-being, and a deeper connection to your own innate healing capacity. This is a time to celebrate the progress you've made, appreciate the journey you've undertaken, and embark on a path
towards sustained health and happiness. Remember, the commitment to self-care extends beyond the Panchakarma

therapies themselves; it's a lifestyle choice that will continue to nourish and support you in the years to come. This is the cornerstone of truly holistic well-being.

Importance of Professional Guidance

Embarking on a Panchakarma journey is a significant commitment to your well-being, a profound step towards restoring balance and vitality within your body and mind. However, the effectiveness and safety of these potent therapies are inextricably linked to the expertise and guidance of a qualified Ayurvedic practitioner. This is not simply a matter of convenience; it's a crucial element ensuring both the efficacy and safety of the process. Choosing the right practitioner is therefore paramount, forming the bedrock of a successful and transformative Panchakarma experience.

The complexity of Panchakarma therapies necessitates a deep understanding of Ayurvedic principles, individual constitution (Prakriti), current imbalances (Vikriti), and the subtle interplay between doshas. A qualified practitioner possesses this comprehensive knowledge, allowing them to tailor the treatment plan to your unique needs, ensuring optimal results while minimizing any potential risks. This individualized approach is central to the efficacy of Panchakarma; a one-size-fits-all approach would be a gross misapplication of this intricate healing system.

Identifying a truly qualified practitioner requires diligence and careful consideration. While the allure of readily available, inexpensive treatments might be tempting, compromising on the quality of care can lead to disappointing, and potentially harmful, outcomes. Remember that Panchakarma therapies are powerful interventions aimed at deep detoxification and rebalancing. Improper application can disrupt delicate bodily systems, potentially causing more harm than good.

The search for a suitable practitioner begins with thorough research. Look for practitioners with a strong educational background in Ayurveda, preferably with advanced training in Panchakarma therapies. Credentials are crucial. Verify their qualifications and certifications, ensuring they've received formal training from reputable institutions. Look for practitioners affiliated with recognized professional organizations, which often have stringent standards for membership and ethical practice.

Online resources, while useful for initial research, should be approached cautiously. Numerous practitioners advertise their services online, but verifying the legitimacy of their claims is essential. Don't solely rely on website testimonials or self-proclaimed expertise. Look for evidence-based information, affiliations with accredited institutions, and perhaps even peer reviews from other healthcare professionals.

Word-of-mouth referrals can be invaluable. If you know someone who has successfully undergone Panchakarma, their personal experience and recommendation can provide invaluable insight. Inquire about their experience with the practitioner, their level of satisfaction with the treatment, and the overall outcome. Such firsthand accounts often offer a more nuanced perspective than generalized online reviews.

During the initial consultation, a thorough assessment of your health history, lifestyle, dietary habits, and current symptoms is crucial. A qualified practitioner will take the time to understand your individual constitution (Prakriti) and identify your current imbalances (Vikriti). They should explain the rationale behind the recommended therapies, detailing the procedures, potential benefits, and potential side effects. Transparency and clear communication are essential indicators of a reputable practitioner.

The consultation should not feel rushed or superficial. A qualified practitioner will answer all your questions thoroughly and patiently, addressing your concerns and clarifying any uncertainties you may have. They will create a personalized treatment plan based on your specific needs and health status, not relying on generic protocols. This individualized approach is the hallmark of a truly effective Panchakarma experience.

Beyond qualifications and credentials, consider the practitioner's approach to patient care. A holistic perspective is vital; true Ayurvedic healing extends beyond the physical body, encompassing the mental, emotional, and spiritual aspects of well-being. The practitioner should demonstrate an understanding of the interconnectedness of these aspects, emphasizing lifestyle modifications alongside the therapies themselves.

The practitioner's ability to integrate Ayurvedic principles with modern medical practices can be a significant advantage. While Ayurveda stands as a complete system of medicine, a collaborative approach with conventional healthcare providers can be beneficial, particularly in managing chronic conditions or addressing specific health concerns. A skilled practitioner will understand when consultation with other healthcare professionals is appropriate and will facilitate seamless communication.

The cost of Panchakarma therapies can vary significantly. While affordability is a factor, remember that choosing a less expensive practitioner simply to save money might jeopardize the safety and efficacy of the treatments. Prioritize quality over cost, understanding that a truly skilled and qualified practitioner will usually command a higher fee due to their experience, knowledge, and the personalized attention they offer. However, it's always advisable to inquire about payment options and any potential financial assistance programs available.

Furthermore, consider the setting of the clinic or treatment center. A clean, comfortable, and serene environment is crucial for relaxation and optimal healing. The facilities should be appropriately equipped to perform the various Panchakarma procedures safely and hygienically. Investigate the practitioner's hygiene practices and adherence to safety protocols.

Remember, embarking on Panchakarma is a commitment to your holistic well-being. Finding a qualified practitioner is not just about finding someone who offers the services; it's about finding a partner in your healing journey, someone who understands your unique needs, and who will guide you with expertise, compassion, and unwavering dedication to your well-being. The time invested in finding the right practitioner is time well spent – an investment that will yield immense returns in terms of your overall health and quality of life. A thorough and diligent search will lay the groundwork for a safe, effective, and transformative Panchakarma experience, paving the way to a healthier, more balanced you. Don't rush this vital decision; your well-being depends on it. The investment in your health is an investment in your future. Take your time, gather information, ask questions, and trust your intuition – you are making a choice that will significantly impact your life's journey.

The process of selecting a qualified Ayurvedic practitioner for Panchakarma is a deeply personal one. It's not just about finding a skilled professional, but also about finding someone with whom you feel comfortable and confident. The therapeutic relationship is a crucial element in the success of Panchakarma, as trust and open communication are essential for a positive and effective treatment experience. Remember, choosing the right practitioner is a key component in maximizing the transformative potential of Panchakarma, setting the stage for a journey towards lasting health and well-being. The results are worth the effort of a careful and considered search. Your well-being is paramount, and your choice of practitioner will directly affect the outcome of your Panchakarma experience.

Ayurvedic Rejuvenation Therapies

Rasayana, a cornerstone of Ayurvedic rejuvenation, transcends the simple notion of extending lifespan. It's a holistic approach focused on enhancing the quality of life, promoting vitality, and fostering a deep sense of well-being that radiates from within. Unlike merely treating illness, Rasayana aims to cultivate a robust constitution capable of resisting disease and aging gracefully. This involves nourishing the body at a fundamental level, strengthening the tissues, sharpening the senses, and enhancing cognitive function. The ultimate goal is to achieve a state of *ojas*, a vital essence embodying radiant health, strength, and immunity.

The principles underlying Rasayana are deeply rooted in the understanding of the body's inherent capacity for self-healing and rejuvenation. Ayurveda posits that our bodies are constantly undergoing processes of creation, maintenance, and decay. While decay is an inevitable part of life, Rasayana aims to optimize the processes of creation and maintenance, slowing down the degenerative process and maximizing the body's inherent longevity. This is achieved through a multi-faceted approach that encompasses dietary modifications, herbal preparations, lifestyle adjustments, and specific therapeutic practices.

Central to Rasayana are the specialized herbal formulations known as *Rasayana Aushadhis*. These potent remedies are meticulously crafted using a combination of herbs, minerals, and sometimes precious metals, carefully selected and combined according to their specific properties and synergistic effects. The selection of herbs is crucial, tailored to the individual's constitution (dosha) and specific needs. A skilled Ayurvedic practitioner plays a vital role in determining the most appropriate Rasayana formulation for an individual. These formulations are not simply a collection of herbs; they are meticulously prepared following traditional methods; often involving complex processes of processing and purification to enhance their potency and bioavailability. This dedication to quality and precision reflects the profound respect Ayurveda holds for the healing power of nature.

Some of the most commonly used Rasayana herbs include:

Ashwagandha (Withania somnifera):
Known as "Indian ginseng," Ashwagandha is an adaptogen that helps the body cope with stress, enhances energy levels, and supports cognitive function. Its rejuvenating properties are widely recognized in Ayurvedic medicine.

Brahmi (Bacopa monnieri):
This herb is renowned for its cognitive-enhancing properties, promoting memory, focus, and mental clarity. It's often used to combat age-related cognitive decline.

Shatavari (Asparagus racemosus):
This herb is
particularly beneficial for women's health, supporting reproductive function and hormone balance. It also possesses rejuvenating properties that contribute to overall well-being.

Amla (Emblica officinalis):
Amla, also known as Indian gooseberry, is a potent antioxidant rich in Vitamin C and other vital nutrients. It's a powerful rejuvenative agent that strengthens the immune system and promotes overall health.

Guduchi (Tinospora cordifolia):
This herb is considered an excellent immunomodulator, helping to strengthen the body's

natural defenses and improve resistance to disease. It also has potent rejuvenating properties.

These herbs, and many others, work synergistically in Rasayana formulations to address various aspects of aging and degeneration. Their combined effects go beyond simply boosting specific physiological functions. They act at a deeper level, promoting overall homeostasis and strengthening the body's ability to maintain its own equilibrium.

However, it is essential to understand that Rasayana is not a quick fix or a magic bullet. It is a long-term commitment to self-care and well-being. The benefits of Rasayana are not immediate; rather, they are cumulative and manifest over time with consistent practice. This long-term approach underscores the holistic philosophy of Ayurveda, which emphasizes the importance of sustainable lifestyle changes rather than relying solely on quick interventions.

Beyond the herbal preparations, Rasayana incorporates a range of lifestyle practices that support the body's natural rejuvenation process. These practices include:

A balanced diet:
Nutrition forms the bedrock of Rasayana. Following a diet that is in accordance with one's dosha, rich in fresh, seasonal fruits and vegetables, whole grains, and legumes, is crucial for providing the body with the necessary nutrients to support its rejuvenation process. Minimizing processed foods, refined sugars, and unhealthy fats is equally important.

Regular exercise:
Moderate physical activity is essential for maintaining physical health and promoting longevity.
Ayurveda recommends a variety of exercise practices, including yoga, pranayama (yogic breathing techniques), and

walking, tailored to the individual's dosha and physical capabilities.

Stress management:
Chronic stress significantly accelerates the aging process. Ayurveda emphasizes the importance of managing stress through practices such as meditation,
mindfulness, and spending time in nature.

Adequate sleep:
Sufficient, restful sleep is vital for cellular repair and rejuvenation. A regular sleep schedule and a calming bedtime routine contribute significantly to the overall success of Rasayana therapies.

Sensory stimulation:
Engaging the senses through activities such as listening to calming music, spending time in nature, or practicing aromatherapy can enhance the overall
experience of Rasayana and promote a sense of well-being.

Positive mental attitude:
A positive mindset and emotional balance are essential for maintaining optimal health and well-being. Practices such as meditation and mindfulness can cultivate a more positive outlook and reduce stress, supporting the rejuvenation process.

The integration of Rasayana into daily life should be gradual and tailored to the individual's needs and preferences. It's not about rigidly following a strict regimen; instead, it's about consciously making choices that support the body's natural ability to heal and rejuvenate. This may involve incorporating specific herbs into the diet, adjusting one's exercise routine, or simply cultivating a more mindful approach to daily life.

Furthermore, it's crucial to emphasize the importance of consulting a qualified Ayurvedic practitioner before embarking on any Rasayana therapy. A personalized approach is vital to ensure that the chosen herbs and practices are appropriate for the individual's constitution and health condition. The practitioner can assess the individual's unique needs, recommend suitable Rasayana formulations, and provide guidance on integrating these therapies into their lifestyle. This collaborative approach ensures the safety and efficacy of the Rasayana regimen, maximizing its benefits and minimizing any potential risks.

In conclusion, Rasayana represents a profound and holistic approach to rejuvenation, offering a path to not only extending lifespan but also enhancing the quality of life. By combining potent herbal remedies with a supportive lifestyle, Rasayana empowers individuals to nurture their bodies and minds, cultivating a state of vibrant health and vitality that extends far beyond the physical realm. It's a journey of self-discovery and empowerment, guiding individuals towards a life characterized by balance, resilience, and lasting well-being. The integration of modern scientific research further validates the efficacy of Rasayana, highlighting its potential as a powerful tool in promoting longevity and overall health. However, the enduring wisdom of Ayurveda remains central, emphasizing the importance of a holistic approach and the essential role of a qualified practitioner in guiding the individual towards their path to rejuvenation.

Key Rasayana Herbs and Their Benefits

Ayurveda's Rasayana therapies utilize a wide array of potent herbs, each contributing unique properties to the overall rejuvenation process. These herbs aren't merely supplements; they are carefully selected and combined to address specific imbalances and strengthen the body's constitution. Understanding their individual benefits allows for a more personalized approach to Rasayana, maximizing its efficacy and tailoring it to individual needs.

Among the most revered Rasayana herbs is **Ashwagandha (Withania somnifera)**, often called the "Indian ginseng." Known for its adaptogenic properties, Ashwagandha helps the body cope with stress, reducing cortisol levels and promoting relaxation. Beyond stress management, it's a powerful nervine tonic, improving cognitive function, memory, and concentration. Studies suggest its potential in boosting immunity and even exhibiting anti-cancer properties. However, it's crucial to note that individual responses may vary, and those with autoimmune conditions should proceed with caution and under the guidance of an Ayurvedic practitioner.

Another keystone herb is **Brahmi (Bacopa monnieri)**, highly regarded for its cognitive-enhancing effects. Traditional Ayurvedic texts describe Brahmi as improving memory, intellect, and overall mental clarity. Modern research corroborates these claims, suggesting Brahmi's potential in improving learning and memory, and even exhibiting neuroprotective effects against age-related cognitive decline. Brahmi's calming properties also make it beneficial for managing anxiety and promoting restful sleep. It's gentle yet powerful, making it suitable for a broad range of individuals, though those on certain medications should consult their physician beforehand.

Gotu Kola (Centella asiatica)
is another remarkable herb with significant Rasayana properties. Traditionally used to improve circulation and cognitive function, Gotu Kola has garnered interest for its potential in wound healing and skin rejuvenation. It's considered a nerve tonic and is thought to promote healthy nerve function and potentially improve memory and mental clarity. Furthermore, Gotu Kola is
believed to support cardiovascular health, promoting healthy blood circulation and reducing inflammation. Its effects are often subtle yet cumulative, gradually improving overall well-being over time.

Shatavari (Asparagus racemosus)
, meaning "the queen of herbs," is highly valued in Ayurveda, particularly for its nourishing and rejuvenating effects on the female
reproductive system. It's renowned for supporting hormonal balance, promoting fertility, and easing menopausal symptoms. Beyond its reproductive benefits, Shatavari is a potent adaptogen, helping the body cope with stress and promoting overall vitality. It's also believed to support digestive health and strengthen the immune system. However, pregnant or breastfeeding women should consult with an Ayurvedic practitioner before using Shatavari.

Amla (Emblica officinalis)
, also known as Indian
gooseberry, is a powerhouse of Vitamin C and other antioxidants. This potent herb is prized for its rejuvenating and immune-boosting properties. It's known to support liver function, enhance digestion, and improve overall gut health. Amla's rich antioxidant profile helps protect cells from damage caused by free radicals, contributing to healthy aging and disease prevention. Its high Vitamin C content

also supports collagen production, contributing to healthy skin and tissue regeneration.

Tulsi (Ocimum tenuiflorum), or holy basil, is a sacred herb in Ayurvedic tradition, revered for its purifying and adaptogenic properties. Its aromatic leaves are used in various preparations to combat stress, improve respiratory function, and boost immunity. Tulsi's powerful antioxidant and anti-inflammatory properties support overall health and well-being, protecting the body from the damaging effects of oxidative stress. Its ability to support respiratory health makes it valuable during seasonal changes and for those prone to respiratory ailments.

Guduchi (Tinospora cordifolia), a potent herb with remarkable adaptogenic and immune-enhancing properties, is known to support the body's natural defense mechanisms. It's often used to enhance immunity, fight infections, and reduce inflammation. Guduchi is particularly effective in supporting detoxification processes, promoting the removal of toxins from the body. Its adaptogenic qualities help the body cope with stress and maintain balance in various bodily systems.

Beyond these individual herbs, the true power of Rasayana often lies in synergistic combinations. Ayurvedic formulations frequently combine multiple herbs, creating potent remedies that address various aspects of health. For instance, a Rasayana formula might combine Ashwagandha for stress management and Brahmi for cognitive enhancement, creating a synergistic effect greater than the sum of its parts. These formulations are often tailored to an individual's unique constitution and specific health goals, requiring the expertise of a qualified Ayurvedic practitioner.

The selection of specific Rasayana herbs and their preparation methods are crucial for optimal efficacy. The quality of the herbs, their processing techniques, and the precise combinations used all play a significant role in determining the overall effectiveness of the Rasayana therapy. Improper preparation or the use of low-quality herbs can diminish their therapeutic value, highlighting the importance of sourcing herbs from reputable suppliers and working with a knowledgeable practitioner.

It's also important to understand that Rasayana is not a quick fix; it's a holistic process that requires commitment and consistency. The benefits of Rasayana are often cumulative, unfolding gradually over time as the body's systems are nourished and strengthened. This process of rejuvenation involves not only the consumption of potent herbal remedies but also the adoption of a supportive lifestyle, including a balanced diet, regular exercise, stress management techniques, and adequate sleep. Furthermore, the integration of yoga and pranayama practices can significantly enhance the effectiveness of Rasayana therapies. The gentle yet effective movements of yoga and the controlled breathing of pranayama help to calm the nervous system, reduce stress, and promote the harmonious flow of prana (vital energy) throughout the body.

The application of Rasayana is deeply personal and should always be guided by a qualified Ayurvedic practitioner. They will assess your unique constitution (Prakriti), identify any imbalances (Vikriti), and recommend the appropriate herbs and formulations to support your specific needs. This personalized approach ensures that the Rasayana therapy aligns with your individual requirements and maximizes its effectiveness. Furthermore, a qualified practitioner can provide guidance on appropriate dosages, preparation methods, potential interactions with other medications, and any precautions that may be necessary.

In conclusion, while the individual benefits of each Rasayana herb are significant, it's the holistic approach and personalized application that truly unlocks the potential of Rasayana for rejuvenation and longevity. The integration of these powerful herbs with a supportive lifestyle, guided by an experienced practitioner, allows individuals to embark on a profound journey toward enhanced well-being, resilience, and a vibrant, fulfilling life. The ancient wisdom of Ayurveda, coupled with modern scientific understanding, offers a powerful path towards achieving optimal health and vitality, extending far beyond the mere extension of lifespan to encompass the richness and quality of life itself. The journey of Rasayana is a testament to the interconnectedness of mind, body, and spirit, highlighting the profound impact of nurturing our inner landscape to cultivate a state of enduring health and well-being.

Lifestyle Practices for Rejuvenation

The profound rejuvenation offered by Rasayana isn't solely reliant on potent herbal formulations. True rejuvenation, as understood within the Ayurvedic framework, necessitates a holistic approach encompassing lifestyle choices that harmonize with the body's natural rhythms and support its inherent healing capacity. These lifestyle practices aren't merely supplementary; they are integral to the success of any Rasayana program, acting as the fertile ground in which the herbal remedies can flourish.

Central to this lifestyle transformation is the mindful cultivation of a balanced diet. While the specific dietary recommendations will vary depending on individual dosha constitution and current imbalances, several overarching principles apply. Emphasis should be placed on consuming fresh, seasonal produce, prioritizing whole, unprocessed foods over refined and packaged items. The six tastes – sweet, sour, salty, bitter, pungent, and astringent – should be incorporated in balanced proportions to avoid any single taste dominating and disrupting the delicate equilibrium. Excessive consumption of any one taste can lead to imbalances, highlighting the importance of mindful eating and awareness of the subtle effects of food on the body. For instance, excessive sweet tastes can aggravate Kapha, while an overabundance of pungent and sour tastes might exacerbate Pitta.

The preparation method of food is equally critical. Ayurveda emphasizes gentle cooking techniques that preserve the nutritional integrity and inherent energies of the ingredients. Steaming, boiling, and slow cooking are preferred over methods that involve excessive heat or harsh processing. The way food is presented also plays a role; eating in a calm, peaceful environment, free from distractions, allows for better digestion and assimilation of nutrients. Mindful eating, paying attention to the textures, aromas, and flavors of the food, promotes satiety and fosters a deeper connection with the nourishment we receive. Regular cleansing practices, such as tongue scraping and oil pulling, further enhance the digestive process, optimizing the body's ability to absorb the vital nutrients essential for rejuvenation.

Physical activity is another cornerstone of the Rasayana lifestyle. However, the type and intensity of exercise should be tailored to individual dosha and physical capacity. Vata individuals, prone to dryness and instability, benefit from gentler, rhythmic exercises like yoga and Tai Chi, avoiding intense or strenuous activities. Pitta individuals, characterized by their fiery nature, might find cooling activities like swimming or walking in nature beneficial, while avoiding overly competitive or stressful physical pursuits. Kapha individuals, who tend towards sluggishness, may benefit from more vigorous exercises like brisk walking, jogging, or cycling to promote circulation and metabolic function. The key is to find an exercise regime that is enjoyable and sustainable, promoting both physical strength and mental clarity without causing undue stress or exhaustion.

Equally important is the management of stress, a significant contributor to aging and depletion of vital energies. Ayurveda offers a variety of techniques to mitigate stress, including meditation, pranayama (yogic breathing exercises), and yoga nidra (yogic sleep). Regular practice of these techniques fosters a state of inner calm and balance, reducing the damaging effects of chronic stress on the body. Spending time in nature, connecting with the earth's energies, is another powerful way to reduce stress and promote emotional well-being. Nature walks, gardening, or simply sitting quietly amidst natural surroundings can be profoundly restorative. Cultivating positive relationships and fostering a sense of community are also essential components of stress management, providing emotional support and a sense of belonging.

Sleep hygiene plays a crucial role in the rejuvenation process. Adequate and restful sleep allows the body to repair and rejuvenate itself, consolidating the benefits of Rasayana therapies and lifestyle changes. Establishing a regular sleep schedule, creating a conducive sleep environment (dark, quiet, and cool), and practicing relaxation techniques before bedtime can significantly improve sleep quality. Avoiding excessive screen time before bed, consuming caffeine and alcohol close to bedtime, and ensuring adequate exposure to sunlight during the day contribute to a more restorative sleep cycle.

In addition to these core practices, other lifestyle adjustments can enhance the effectiveness of the Rasayana journey. These include maintaining good personal hygiene, practicing self-massage (Abhyanga) with warm, medicated oils appropriate to the individual's dosha, and cultivating a sense of purpose and meaning in life. Engaging in activities that bring joy and fulfillment, fostering social connections, and pursuing creative endeavors are all valuable aspects of a Rasayana lifestyle, contributing to overall well-being and longevity.

The Rasayana approach is not merely about extending lifespan; it's about enhancing the quality of life, fostering vitality, resilience, and a profound sense of well-being. It's about cultivating a vibrant, fulfilling existence characterized by clarity, energy, and a deep connection with oneself and the world around. By integrating these lifestyle practices with the judicious use of Rasayana herbs and the guidance of an experienced Ayurvedic practitioner, individuals can embark on a transformative journey toward optimal health, enduring vitality, and a truly rejuvenated life. Remember that this journey is a personal one, requiring patience, consistency, and a commitment to self-care. The rewards, however, far outweigh the effort, leading to a life characterized by increased energy, enhanced mental clarity, improved physical resilience, and a profound sense of inner peace and well-being. The ancient wisdom of Ayurveda, when implemented thoughtfully and consistently, offers a pathway to a life lived not just longer, but richer and more meaningful. This integration of herbal remedies and lifestyle changes constitutes the true essence of Rasayana – a holistic approach to rejuvenation that nourishes the body, mind, and spirit, fostering a state of enduring health and vitality that extends far beyond mere physical longevity. It is a journey of self-discovery, a profound connection to one's inner self, and a harmonious integration with the natural world, ultimately leading to a truly rejuvenated and fulfilling life.

Practical Tips

The journey toward rejuvenation through Rasayana is a deeply personal one, a continuous process of refinement and adaptation. While potent herbal formulations play a vital role, their efficacy is significantly amplified when interwoven with a daily lifestyle that fosters balance and harmony within the body. This integration isn't a rigid regimen, but rather a flexible framework, adaptable to individual needs and preferences. The key lies in consistency and mindful attention to the details that cumulatively contribute to overall well-being.

One of the most fundamental aspects is establishing a consistent daily routine, or Dinacharya. This isn't about strict adherence to a timetable, but rather about creating a predictable structure that supports the body's natural rhythms. Waking before sunrise, ideally around 6 am, allows you to harness the invigorating energy of the morning. This is a time for gentle cleansing, such as tongue scraping and oil pulling, followed by a warm cup of herbal tea or water infused with lemon and ginger. These practices aid in detoxification and stimulate digestion, preparing the body for the day ahead. The early morning hours are also ideal for practicing yoga or meditation, setting a positive tone for the day and nurturing both physical and mental well-being.

Nutrition plays a pivotal role in supporting the Rasayana process. While specific dietary recommendations vary based on individual dosha constitution, the overarching principles emphasize whole, unprocessed foods. Prioritizing seasonal fruits and vegetables, locally sourced whenever possible, ensures the intake of nutrient-rich, easily digestible foods. Incorporating a wide array of colors into your meals maximizes the range of phytochemicals and antioxidants consumed. Regular consumption of ghee (clarified butter), in moderation, is highly recommended for its nourishing qualities and its ability to support the absorption of fat-soluble vitamins. Spices such as turmeric, ginger, and cinnamon, known for their anti-inflammatory and antioxidant properties, should be liberally incorporated into your diet. Careful attention should be paid to mindful eating, savoring each bite and avoiding distractions that might hinder proper digestion.

Beyond diet, maintaining optimal hydration is crucial for all bodily functions, including the efficient absorption and utilization of Rasayana herbs. Water, ideally purified or filtered, should be consumed throughout the day, especially between meals rather than during meals. Incorporating herbal infusions such as ginger tea or fennel tea aids in digestion and can enhance the detoxification process. Avoiding excessive caffeine and alcohol is important, as these substances can disrupt the delicate balance sought through Rasayana practices.

Sleep is another cornerstone of the Rasayana lifestyle. Adequate, restorative sleep is essential for cellular repair and rejuvenation. Aim for 7-8 hours of uninterrupted sleep each night, maintaining a regular sleep schedule to support the body's natural circadian rhythms. Creating a relaxing bedtime routine, such as taking a warm bath or reading a book, helps in preparing the mind and body for restful sleep. Avoiding screen time before bed is essential, as the blue light emitted by electronic devices can interfere with melatonin production, impacting sleep quality.

Stress management forms an integral part of Rasayana. Chronic stress can deplete the body's resources, hindering the effectiveness of any rejuvenation program. Regular practice of stress-reducing techniques, such as yoga, meditation, pranayama (breathing exercises), or spending time in nature, are essential. Incorporating mindfulness practices into daily life, such as paying attention to your breath during routine activities, helps in cultivating a sense of presence and reducing the impact of daily stressors. Seeking support from a therapist or counselor can be immensely beneficial in managing chronic stress.

Regular physical activity is also crucial. The type and intensity of exercise should be tailored to your individual dosha and physical capabilities. Gentle forms of exercise, such as walking, yoga, or tai chi, are generally recommended. The goal is to promote circulation, improve lymphatic drainage, and reduce stress levels without overexerting the body. Finding an activity that you enjoy and that fits into your lifestyle is essential for long-term adherence.

Finally, fostering positive social connections and engaging in activities that bring joy and fulfillment are also vital components of a Rasayana lifestyle. Strong social support networks provide emotional resilience and reduce the burden of stress. Cultivating hobbies and activities that provide a sense of purpose and satisfaction enhances overall well-being and strengthens one's ability to cope with adversity.

Integrating Rasayana into daily life is not about drastic changes but about subtle shifts in lifestyle, a gradual and conscious integration of practices that support the body's natural healing capacity. By incorporating these practical tips into your routine, you can lay the foundation for a life of vibrant health, vitality, and long-term well-being, transforming the pursuit of rejuvenation into a joyful and fulfilling journey. The continuous refinement and adaptation of these practices based on individual experiences will lead to a profound sense of self-awareness and a deeply enriching connection to one's inner self and the natural world. This is the true essence of Rasayana—a holistic approach to rejuvenation that transcends mere longevity and embraces a truly vibrant and fulfilling existence.

Remember, consistency is key. Small, consistent changes over time yield far greater results than sporadic bursts of intense effort. Don't be discouraged by occasional setbacks; view them as opportunities for learning and refinement. The journey towards rejuvenation is a marathon, not a sprint, and it's a journey best undertaken with patience, self-compassion, and a deep commitment to nurturing your mind, body, and spirit. Seek the guidance of a qualified Ayurvedic practitioner to tailor a Rasayana program specifically designed to meet your individual needs and constitution. Their expertise will help you navigate the nuances of herbal formulations and lifestyle modifications, ensuring a safe and effective path towards rejuvenation and sustained well-being. Embrace the wisdom of Ayurveda, and embark on this transformative journey towards a life of enduring vitality and profound inner peace.

Furthermore, consider incorporating journaling into your daily routine. Reflecting on your experiences, both physical and emotional, can provide valuable insights into your individual needs and responses to different practices. This ongoing self-assessment allows for greater adaptability and personalization of your Rasayana program. Note any changes in your energy levels, sleep quality, digestion, and overall mood. Track your food intake and the effects of different herbs and spices. Document your yoga practice and other activities. This ongoing record becomes a powerful tool for self-understanding, enabling you to refine your approach and optimize your journey towards rejuvenation.

Finally, remember that Rasayana is not a quick fix, but a lifelong commitment to self-care and holistic well-being. It's a pathway to cultivate a deep connection with your body and its inherent wisdom, nurturing its innate capacity for healing and rejuvenation. Embrace this journey with patience, consistency, and a deep appreciation for the ancient wisdom of Ayurveda. The rewards – a life of vibrant health, enduring vitality, and profound inner peace – far surpass any temporary discomfort or challenges along the way. The ancient art of Rasayana offers a path towards a truly fulfilling and meaningful life, not just a longer one. Embrace this path, and allow the wisdom of Ayurveda to guide you on your journey towards lasting rejuvenation.

Research and Evidence

The profound claims of Rasayana, promising rejuvenation and extended lifespan, naturally invite scrutiny from a modern scientific perspective. While the traditional Ayurvedic understanding of Rasayana relies on holistic principles and centuries of empirical observation, the burgeoning field of scientific research is beginning to unveil the mechanisms behind its efficacy. This exploration is not about replacing the ancient wisdom with a purely reductionist approach, but rather about integrating modern scientific understanding to enhance our appreciation and application of Rasayana principles.

One crucial area of investigation focuses on the phytochemical composition of Rasayana herbs. Many of these herbs, such as Ashwagandha (Withania somnifera), Amalaki (Emblica officinalis), and Shatavari (Asparagus racemosus), have been subjected to rigorous phytochemical analysis, revealing a complex array of bioactive compounds. These include various antioxidants, such as polyphenols and flavonoids, which combat oxidative stress, a key contributor to aging and age-related diseases. Studies have demonstrated the potent antioxidant capacity of these compounds, suggesting a mechanism by which Rasayana herbs may contribute to cellular protection and longevity. For example, research on Amalaki has revealed its remarkable ability to scavenge free radicals, protecting against DNA damage and cellular senescence. Similarly, Ashwagandha extracts have shown significant antioxidant and anti-inflammatory properties in various in vitro and in vivo studies, suggesting their potential role in mitigating age-related inflammation, a pervasive factor in the development of chronic diseases.

Beyond antioxidant activity, Rasayana herbs often exhibit other bioactive properties relevant to rejuvenation. Some possess adaptogenic qualities, meaning they help the body adapt to stress. Ashwagandha, for instance, is well-known for its adaptogenic effects, reducing cortisol levels and improving stress resilience. This is particularly relevant in the context of Rasayana, as chronic stress is a significant accelerant of aging. By promoting stress resilience, Rasayana herbs may indirectly contribute to longevity by mitigating the detrimental effects of stress on the body.

Another significant aspect of Rasayana is its impact on the immune system. Many Rasayana herbs possess immunomodulatory properties, meaning they can modulate and enhance the body's immune response. This is crucial as the immune system weakens with age, increasing susceptibility to infections and diseases. Research on herbs like Tulsi (Ocimum tenuiflorum) and Guduchi (Tinospora cordifolia) suggests their ability to stimulate immune function, enhancing the body's ability to fight off infections and potentially reducing the incidence of age-related immune decline.

The impact of Rasayana on neuroprotection is also attracting significant scientific attention. Several studies suggest that certain Rasayana herbs can enhance cognitive function and protect against neurodegenerative diseases. For example, research on Brahmi (Bacopa monnieri) indicates its potential to improve memory and cognitive performance, possibly by influencing neurotransmitter levels and promoting neurogenesis. These findings highlight the potential of Rasayana herbs in maintaining brain health and delaying age-related cognitive decline.

However, it's crucial to acknowledge that much of the scientific research on Rasayana is still in its early stages.

Many studies are conducted in vitro or on animal models, and more robust clinical trials are needed to fully validate the claims of Rasayana's rejuvenating effects on humans. Furthermore, the complex interplay of various herbs within traditional Rasayana formulations presents a challenge to scientific investigation, as isolating the effects of individual components can be difficult. The synergistic effects of the combined herbs may be more potent than the sum of their individual parts, a phenomenon that requires further research to fully understand.

The challenges in translating the traditional Ayurvedic understanding of Rasayana into the language of modern science underscore the need for a holistic approach. While scientific research is essential for validating the efficacy of Rasayana herbs and practices, it's equally important to acknowledge the limitations of a purely reductionist approach. The traditional Ayurvedic perspective emphasizes the interconnectedness of mind, body, and spirit, and the impact of lifestyle factors on overall well-being. Rasayana, therefore, cannot be understood solely through the lens of isolated biochemical pathways.

To fully appreciate the benefits of Rasayana, it's crucial to consider the entire framework of Ayurvedic principles. This includes maintaining a balanced diet tailored to one's individual dosha, incorporating regular exercise such as yoga and pranayama, practicing mindfulness and stress-reduction techniques, and fostering a positive mental attitude. These lifestyle practices are integral to the effectiveness of Rasayana therapies, creating a synergistic effect that transcends the impact of herbal formulations alone. In essence, Rasayana is not merely about consuming specific herbs; it's about embracing a holistic lifestyle that promotes balance, harmony, and vitality at all levels.

The integration of Ayurvedic principles with modern scientific methodology holds immense promise for advancing our understanding of health, aging, and longevity. By combining the wisdom of traditional medicine with the rigor of scientific research, we can unlock the full potential of Rasayana and develop innovative strategies for promoting healthy aging and extending lifespan. This requires collaborative efforts between Ayurvedic practitioners, scientists, and researchers, fostering interdisciplinary collaborations that bridge the gap between ancient wisdom and modern scientific inquiry.

The future of Rasayana research will likely involve a more nuanced approach, incorporating advanced technologies such as metabolomics and genomics to better understand the intricate interactions between Rasayana herbs and the human body. This integrated approach could help identify specific biomarkers associated with Rasayana's effects, allowing for more precise assessments of its efficacy and safety. Furthermore, personalized approaches tailored to individual genetic predispositions and doshic constitutions are likely to become increasingly important, ensuring that Rasayana therapies are optimized for maximum individual benefit.

In conclusion, while the scientific evidence supporting the rejuvenating effects of Rasayana is still emerging, the promising findings from existing research warrant further investigation. The potent antioxidant, adaptogenic, immunomodulatory, and neuroprotective properties of many Rasayana herbs suggest their potential to significantly impact healthy aging and longevity. However, it is crucial to remember that Rasayana is not a panacea, but rather a holistic approach that requires a commitment to a balanced lifestyle, mindful practices, and a profound respect for the intricate wisdom of Ayurveda. The path to rejuvenation, as revealed by Rasayana, is a journey of self-discovery and mindful self-care, a continuous process of refinement and adaptation that leads to a life of vibrant health, enduring vitality, and profound inner peace. The future integration of traditional Ayurvedic knowledge with the advancements of modern science promises to unlock even greater understanding and application of this ancient art of rejuvenation. The journey is long, but the rewards, a life of health and vitality, are well worth the effort.

The Digestive Fire

Agni, the Sanskrit word for "fire," represents the digestive fire within each of us. In Ayurveda, Agni is not merely a physiological process; it's a vital force, a transformative energy that fuels our very existence. It's the powerhouse responsible for breaking down food, extracting nutrients, and eliminating waste. A robust Agni ensures efficient metabolism, clear skin, stable energy levels, and a sharp mind. Conversely, a weakened Agni, often referred to as *mandagni*
, leads to a cascade of imbalances that manifest as a variety of health concerns. Understanding Agni and
nurturing its strength is paramount to achieving optimal digestive health and overall well-being within the Ayurvedic framework.

The strength of your Agni is deeply personal and fluctuates based on a multitude of internal and external factors. While genetics play a role in determining your inherent digestive capacity, lifestyle choices significantly impact Agni's vitality. Stress, irregular eating patterns, poor food combinations, insufficient sleep, and emotional imbalances all contribute to a weakening of this essential metabolic fire. Conversely, consistent healthy habits, balanced nutrition, and mindful practices nurture a strong and efficient Agni.

Think of Agni as a carefully tended flame. A roaring bonfire requires consistent fuel of the right kind, sufficient oxygen, and a stable environment. Similarly, a strong Agni thrives on wholesome, easily digestible foods, appropriate cooking methods, and a relaxed, balanced lifestyle. Conversely, a dwindling ember responds poorly to erratic feeding, improper food combinations, and constant stress. The quality and timing of meals play a critical role. Consuming large quantities of food, especially late at night, overwhelms Agni, hindering its ability to efficiently process the incoming nutrients. Conversely, eating small, frequent meals allows for consistent digestive activity and prevents overburdening the system.

The Ayurvedic system identifies six tastes – sweet, sour, salty, pungent, bitter, and astringent – each playing a unique role in supporting or hindering Agni. A balanced diet encompassing all six tastes, customized to your individual dosha, optimally fuels your digestive fire. However, even the most balanced diet can falter if not prepared and consumed correctly. Cold foods and drinks, particularly immediately before or after a meal, are known to dampen Agni's vigor. Similarly, mixing incompatible food groups can lead to sluggish digestion and the accumulation of ama.

The time of day also influences Agni's strength. According to Ayurvedic principles, Agni is at its peak during midday, gradually waning as the day progresses. Therefore, the largest and most substantial meal is traditionally recommended during midday, followed by lighter meals in the afternoon and evening. The concept of digestive rhythm is crucial. Consistent mealtimes help regulate Agni's activity, paving the way for consistent and optimal digestion.

Beyond diet, several lifestyle factors influence Agni's strength. Chronic stress significantly weakens Agni, diverting energy away from digestion and towards the body's stress response mechanism. Insufficient sleep further diminishes Agni's strength. Ayurveda emphasizes the importance of consistent, restful sleep of approximately seven to eight hours to support digestive function. Regular exercise, tailored to your dosha, stimulates Agni by improving blood flow and metabolic activity. Excessive physical activity, however, can overtax the system, weakening Agni. The key is finding a balance that promotes physical health without excessive exertion.

Beyond the physical elements, mental and emotional well-being significantly impact Agni. Chronic anxiety, worry, and anger are known to hinder digestion. Mindful eating practices, such as savoring each bite, chewing thoroughly, and eating in a peaceful environment, nurture Agni's strength. Conversely, rushed meals, distracted eating, and negative emotions during meals diminish Agni's efficiency.

Recognizing the signs of weak Agni is crucial for early intervention. Common symptoms include indigestion, bloating, gas, constipation, diarrhea, heartburn, acid reflux, fatigue, food cravings, and skin problems. If left unaddressed, these digestive imbalances can manifest into more serious health issues. These symptoms are often subtle and can easily be overlooked. Observing the consistency of your bowel movements, the timing and degree of satiety after eating, and any feelings of sluggishness or heaviness after a meal can help gauge the status of your Agni.

In addition to dietary and lifestyle modifications, various Ayurvedic therapies can strengthen Agni. Herbal remedies, tailored to individual needs and doshas, play a significant role in supporting digestion. Ginger, turmeric, fennel seeds, and coriander are commonly used to stimulate Agni and alleviate digestive distress. However, it is crucial to consult a qualified Ayurvedic practitioner for personalized recommendations. Self-treating can lead to undesirable consequences.

Panchakarma, a comprehensive Ayurvedic detoxification program, can be highly beneficial for restoring balanced digestive function. This holistic approach, under the guidance of an experienced practitioner, aims to cleanse the body of accumulated ama and restore Agni's strength. However, it's crucial to remember that Panchakarma is a rigorous process and shouldn't be undertaken lightly. Proper guidance and supervision are paramount for safety and efficacy.

Ultimately, nurturing Agni is an ongoing process that requires consistent attention and commitment to healthy habits. It's not a quick fix but a gradual cultivation of balance and well-being. By understanding the factors influencing Agni's strength and implementing the necessary adjustments, you pave the way for optimal digestion, enhanced nutrient absorption, improved energy levels, a clear mind, and a healthier, more vibrant life. This is the cornerstone of
Ayurvedic health—a holistic approach that integrates mind, body, and spirit to create a symphony of balanced vitality. The journey to a stronger Agni requires patience, self-awareness, and a commitment to nurturing your inner fire. The rewards, however, are immeasurable, leading to a state of profound well-being that radiates from the inside out. It's about fostering a harmonious relationship with your body, respecting its rhythms, and honoring its innate wisdom. This understanding underpins the entire Ayurvedic philosophy, guiding you towards a path of lasting health and well-being. Remember that consulting with a qualified Ayurvedic practitioner is essential for personalized guidance and to address any specific digestive issues you may be experiencing. They can provide tailored recommendations based on your unique constitution, lifestyle, and health history.

Undigested Food and Toxins

The foundation of Ayurvedic health, as we've explored, rests on the strength of Agni, the digestive fire. However, a robust Agni alone isn't sufficient to guarantee optimal health. The presence or absence of *ama*, the Sanskrit term for undigested food and accumulated toxins, plays an equally crucial role. Ama is not simply leftover food particles; it's a complex byproduct of impaired digestion that can significantly impact every aspect of your well-being.

Imagine your digestive system as a finely tuned engine. When Agni is strong and functioning optimally, food is efficiently broken down, nutrients are absorbed, and waste products are eliminated smoothly. However, when Agni is weakened—due to factors like poor dietary choices, stress, irregular eating habits, or insufficient sleep—the digestive process becomes sluggish. Food isn't fully digested, leading to the formation of ama. This ama, instead of being expelled, accumulates in the body, clinging to tissues and organs, clouding the channels (srotas) that govern the flow of energy and nutrients throughout the system.

Ama manifests in various forms. It's not always easily identifiable as a single, distinct substance. Instead, its presence reveals itself through a constellation of symptoms, often subtle at first but progressively worsening if left unaddressed. These can include sluggish digestion, bloating, gas, constipation, or diarrhea. The quality of ama varies depending on the individual's constitution (Prakriti), their dietary habits, and the nature of the undigested food. For instance, someone with a predominantly Kapha constitution might experience heavier, more mucus-like ama, while a Pitta individual might see more inflammatory manifestations. This explains why Ayurvedic treatment is personalized, accounting for individual differences.

The impact of ama extends far beyond digestive discomfort. Its accumulation acts as a barrier, hindering the efficient absorption of nutrients. This nutrient deficiency can manifest as fatigue, low energy levels, weakened immunity, and even skin problems like acne or eczema. Furthermore, ama can obstruct the flow of prana (vital energy) throughout the body, contributing to a general sense of sluggishness, mental fog, and difficulty concentrating. Over time, chronic ama accumulation can contribute to the development of more serious health conditions, emphasizing the importance of early intervention and preventative measures.

Recognizing ama involves a holistic assessment. There's no single test to identify ama, but rather a collection of observations that point towards its presence. These indicators range from the obvious—like persistent digestive issues—to the more subtle, such as a coated tongue, bad breath, changes in body odor, or a dull complexion. A coated tongue, for instance, is a classic sign. The coating's color and texture can offer clues about the type of ama present. A thick, white coating often suggests a Kapha imbalance, while a yellow coating may indicate Pitta aggravation. Similarly, a change in your usual body odor or a persistent unpleasant breath can signal the body's struggle to eliminate toxins effectively. These seemingly minor details are valuable insights into the body's inner workings, highlighting the need for attentive self-observation.

Further signs of ama accumulation can be seen in subtle changes in mental clarity. If you're experiencing persistent brain fog, poor concentration, or difficulty making decisions, it could be an indication of ama interfering with the smooth flow of prana. Similarly, if your skin appears dull, lifeless, or prone to breakouts despite seemingly following a healthy diet and skincare regimen, it could be a sign of toxins attempting to escape through the skin. This emphasizes the interconnectedness of systems in Ayurveda—skin issues often reflect internal imbalances. Finally, chronic fatigue, unexplained weight gain or loss, and persistent aches and pains can also be subtle indicators.

The key to recognizing ama is to pay close attention to your body's signals. Regular self-observation is crucial. Observe your digestion after every meal; are you experiencing any discomfort, bloating, or heaviness? Note the color and consistency of your stools; are they well-formed, or is there an indication of undigested food? Consider the clarity of your mind; is it sharp and focused, or clouded and sluggish? Become acutely aware of the subtle changes within your body. This level of self-awareness is fundamental to preventing the accumulation of ama and maintaining overall well-being.

Furthermore, the process of identifying ama is not solely based on subjective observations; objective assessment plays a vital role. An Ayurvedic practitioner, through a detailed examination, can gather valuable insights. They would examine your pulse (nadi pariksha), assess your tongue, observe your skin, inquire about your bowel habits, and assess your overall energy levels. This comprehensive assessment provides a much more thorough picture than any single indicator, allowing for a personalized diagnosis and treatment plan. Through this process, they can determine not only the presence of ama, but also its location, type, and underlying cause. This underscores the importance of seeking guidance from a qualified Ayurvedic professional for accurate assessment and tailored solutions.

Beyond the individual symptoms, there's a broader pattern to recognize. If you're experiencing a cluster of these symptoms—digestive issues, mental fog, skin problems, unexplained fatigue—it strongly suggests the presence of ama. This accumulation isn't merely a symptom itself; it's a significant factor that exacerbates other imbalances. For example, ama can further weaken Agni, creating a vicious cycle of impaired digestion and toxin buildup. Addressing the root cause, which in this scenario is the ama, is vital for breaking this cycle and restoring balance.

Understanding ama is not just about recognizing symptoms; it's about understanding the root causes. While poor digestion is the primary driver, several lifestyle factors contribute to its formation. These include consuming excessive amounts of processed foods, heavy or difficult-to-digest foods, and cold or raw foods, especially when your Agni is weak. Additionally, stress, lack of sleep, emotional imbalances, and insufficient physical activity can all negatively impact digestion and contribute to the accumulation of ama. These factors are intertwined and often exacerbate each other. For example, stress not only weakens Agni but also often leads to poor dietary choices, further hindering digestion. Similarly, lack of sleep can impair the body's natural detoxification processes.

Once you've identified potential signs of ama, the next step involves addressing the issue through a multifaceted approach. This is where the wisdom of Ayurveda shines, offering a holistic solution that goes beyond simply treating symptoms. The Ayurvedic approach emphasizes gentle yet powerful techniques aimed at promoting optimal digestion, eliminating toxins, and restoring balance. These include dietary changes, lifestyle modifications, and potentially, Ayurvedic detoxification therapies (Panchakarma). Dietary modifications are crucial. This involves focusing on easily digestible foods, incorporating spices that aid digestion, and reducing the consumption of processed foods, refined sugars, and overly rich or heavy meals. The specific dietary recommendations will depend on your individual constitution (Prakriti) and the type of ama present. A qualified Ayurvedic practitioner will be able to provide personalized guidance.

Similarly, lifestyle modifications play a vital role. This involves prioritizing regular exercise, incorporating stress-reducing techniques like meditation or yoga, ensuring adequate sleep, and maintaining a balanced daily routine (Dinacharya). These lifestyle adjustments aren't just about addressing symptoms; they are fundamental to creating an environment where the body can effectively cleanse itself and prevent the further accumulation of ama. Incorporating practices like regular self-massage (Abhyanga) can also promote lymphatic drainage and toxin elimination. This holistic perspective emphasizes the interplay between diet, lifestyle, and overall well-being.

In cases of significant ama accumulation, Ayurvedic detoxification therapies (Panchakarma) may be recommended. These therapies are supervised by experienced practitioners and are tailored to the individual's constitution and condition. They involve a series of procedures, such as oil massages (Abhyanga), herbal steam treatments (Swedana), and specialized cleansing techniques, all aimed at gently removing ama from the body's tissues and channels. However, it's crucial to emphasize that Panchakarma should only be undertaken under the guidance of a qualified Ayurvedic practitioner. These therapies are potent and require expertise to ensure safety and efficacy.

The journey to eliminating ama and restoring digestive health is a process, not a quick fix. It demands patience, self-awareness, and a commitment to healthy lifestyle choices. By understanding the role of ama in your overall well-being, you can take proactive steps to prevent its accumulation and promote a state of vibrant health. Remember, Ayurveda offers a holistic pathway to achieving optimal health, not just through treating symptoms but by addressing the root causes and fostering a balanced relationship with your body. With consistent effort and personalized guidance, you can pave the way for a healthier, more energized, and more balanced life.

Dietary Strategies for Improving Digestion

The cornerstone of Ayurvedic digestion lies in understanding and nurturing Agni, your digestive fire. However, even with a robust Agni, certain dietary choices can hinder the digestive process, leading to the accumulation of ama. Therefore, focusing on dietary strategies is paramount in improving digestion and preventing ama formation. This involves careful consideration of food combinations, cooking methods, and mindful eating practices.

One of the most crucial aspects of Ayurvedic dietary advice is the principle of food combining. Certain food combinations are considered harmonious, promoting efficient digestion, while others can create digestive disharmony and ama buildup. For instance, combining heavy proteins (like meat or dairy) with starchy carbohydrates (like rice or potatoes) can be particularly challenging for the digestive system. The reason for this lies in the different digestive enzymes required to break down these food groups. Simultaneous digestion of these disparate foods can overload the system, leading to sluggish digestion and fermentation, ultimately producing ama.

Instead, Ayurveda recommends consuming protein-rich foods with lighter vegetables or salads. Similarly, combining starchy carbohydrates with easily digestible vegetables is more beneficial. For example, a meal of kitchari (a nourishing Ayurvedic dish made from rice and lentils) with steamed greens is easier to digest than a meal of rice and lentils followed by a large portion of red meat. This careful pairing of foods allows the body to efficiently allocate its digestive resources, ensuring optimal nutrient absorption and minimizing ama formation.

Beyond food combinations, the way food is prepared greatly influences its digestibility. Ayurveda emphasizes the use of simple cooking methods that preserve the natural nutrients and energy of the food. Overcooked foods, particularly those that are burnt or charred, are more difficult to digest and can create ama. The high temperatures involved in these cooking methods can disrupt the delicate balance of nutrients within the food, diminishing its nutritional value and increasing its potential to create ama.

Steaming, boiling, and gentle sautéing are preferred methods in Ayurveda, as these preserve the integrity of the food and make it more readily digestible. Furthermore, the use of fresh, seasonal produce is always encouraged. Seasonal foods are not only at their nutritional peak but are also more in tune with the body's natural rhythms and needs. The taste and texture of seasonal foods align with the current doshic balance, making them more easily digestible and less likely to create ama.

The importance of spices in promoting digestion shouldn't be overlooked. Ayurvedic cuisine is renowned for its flavorful use of spices that aid in digestion. Ginger, turmeric, cumin, coriander, and fennel are just a few examples of spices that stimulate Agni and improve the efficiency of the digestive process. These spices contain active compounds with anti-inflammatory and carminative properties, which help prevent gas, bloating, and other digestive discomforts. They also possess antibacterial and antimicrobial properties. Adding these spices to your meals can significantly improve digestion and reduce ama formation.

Mindful eating is an integral part of Ayurvedic dietary recommendations. This goes beyond simply choosing the right foods; it involves being fully present during meals.

Eating in a rushed or distracted state can interfere with proper digestion. The brain's digestive process begins even before the food touches your tongue, with the sensory experience—the smell, sight, and anticipation—triggering the release of digestive enzymes. When you eat in a hurried and stressed manner, this process is interrupted, weakening your Agni.

To promote mindful eating, Ayurveda suggests that you eat in a calm and relaxed atmosphere. Chewing your food thoroughly is essential, as this initiates the digestive process in the mouth. Adequate chewing increases the surface area of the food, making it easier for enzymes to break it down, reducing the workload on your stomach and intestines. This meticulous approach to eating reduces the potential for ama formation.

Furthermore, Ayurveda emphasizes the importance of maintaining a regular eating schedule. Eating at approximately the same times each day helps regulate your digestive rhythms, improving the efficiency of your digestive system. Inconsistent eating patterns can disrupt Agni, leading to poor digestion and the accumulation of ama. By setting consistent meal times, you help your body anticipate the digestive process, leading to better nutrient absorption and less chance of ama formation.

Portion control also plays a significant role in maintaining digestive health. Overeating places unnecessary stress on the digestive system. It's better to eat smaller meals more frequently, allowing your digestive system to work efficiently without being overwhelmed. This approach aligns with the Ayurvedic principle of moderation, suggesting that balance is crucial for optimal health. Excessive quantities of food can easily lead to ama.

The six tastes (rasa) in Ayurveda—sweet, sour, salty, bitter, pungent, and astringent—each play a role in digestion and overall health. While all six tastes are necessary for a balanced diet, understanding their effects on Agni is crucial.
Sweet tastes are generally considered grounding and nourishing but can be difficult to digest in excess. Sour tastes help to stimulate Agni, while salty tastes can help in digestion and the absorption of nutrients. Bitter tastes support detoxification and liver function, while pungent tastes stimulate Agni and promote the elimination of toxins. Astringent tastes are useful in balancing excess and support the elimination of ama. A balanced diet incorporating all six tastes in moderation promotes optimal digestion and minimizes the risk of ama formation.

It is important to note that dietary recommendations in Ayurveda are highly personalized. What works for one individual might not work for another, as each person's constitution (prakriti) and current state of health are unique. A qualified Ayurvedic practitioner can assess your individual dosha and current health status to create a personalized
dietary plan tailored to your specific needs.

The elimination of ama isn't simply about consuming specific foods; it involves a holistic approach to lifestyle. Coupling dietary modifications with other Ayurvedic practices, such as yoga, meditation, and stress management techniques, amplifies the beneficial effects of these dietary changes. By adopting a comprehensive approach that addresses the mind, body, and spirit, you enhance your body's ability to digest food efficiently and eliminate ama effectively. Remember that the journey to improved digestion and optimal health is a gradual process that requires patience, consistency, and self-awareness. With a combination of mindful dietary choices and other Ayurvedic practices, you can restore balance, strengthen your Agni, and pave the way for a healthier, more energized you. Regular consultation with an Ayurvedic practitioner will provide guidance specific to your individual needs, ensuring that you're on the right path towards optimal digestive health.

Herbal Remedies for Digestive Issues

Building upon the foundation of mindful eating and lifestyle practices, we now delve into the rich treasure trove of Ayurvedic herbal remedies that can significantly enhance digestive health. Ayurveda recognizes the intricate relationship between the digestive system and overall well-being, understanding that imbalances in digestion can manifest as various health concerns. These herbal remedies, when used correctly and under the guidance of a qualified practitioner, can effectively address specific digestive issues, supporting the body's natural healing processes. It's crucial to remember that these are not standalone solutions; they work best in conjunction with the dietary and lifestyle adjustments discussed previously.

One of the most commonly used herbs in Ayurveda for digestive support is ginger (
Zingiber officinale
). Its pungent and warming nature helps stimulate Agni, the digestive fire, promoting efficient breakdown and assimilation of food.
Ginger is particularly beneficial for relieving nausea, gas, and bloating, common symptoms of sluggish digestion. It can be consumed in various forms, including fresh ginger juice, ginger tea, or powdered ginger added to meals. For those experiencing nausea, a small piece of fresh ginger can be sucked on throughout the day. Ginger tea, prepared by steeping fresh ginger slices in hot water, offers a soothing and comforting effect. However, those with Pitta dosha should consume ginger in moderation, as its intense heating properties can aggravate Pitta imbalances.

Another powerful digestive herb is turmeric (
Curcuma longa
). The active compound in turmeric, curcumin, possesses potent anti-inflammatory and antioxidant

properties. It helps reduce inflammation in the digestive tract, alleviating symptoms like heartburn, indigestion, and irritable bowel syndrome (IBS). Turmeric also aids in liver detoxification, which is crucial for efficient digestion and nutrient absorption. It can be added to curries, soups, or taken as a supplement, often in conjunction with black pepper to enhance its bioavailability. For those with Kapha dosha, incorporating turmeric into the diet can be particularly beneficial in supporting the digestive system's efficiency.

Triphala, a potent Ayurvedic formulation composed of three fruits – Amalaki (Indian gooseberry), Bibhitaki, and Haritaki– is renowned for its remarkable ability to cleanse and
rejuvenate the digestive system. It gently stimulates bowel movements, helping to eliminate toxins and waste products from the gut. Triphala also possesses astringent properties, helping to improve gut lining integrity. It's often used to address constipation, improve gut flora, and support overall digestive health. However, it is recommended to use Triphala under the guidance of an Ayurvedic practitioner, especially for those with sensitive digestive systems, as its potency can lead to loose stools if taken excessively. Taking it before bed can help with regular morning bowel movements.

For those struggling with gas and bloating, fennel (*Foeniculum vulgare*) seeds are a time-honored remedy.
Their carminative properties help to relax the abdominal muscles, relieving discomfort and promoting the expulsion of trapped gas. Fennel seeds can be chewed after meals or steeped as a tea. Their mild, sweet flavor makes them a palatable choice for those seeking a gentle yet effective digestive aid. Fennel is considered generally safe for all doshas, making it a versatile option for various digestive concerns. Combining fennel with other carminative herbs, such as coriander and cumin, can enhance its effectiveness.

Cumin (*Cuminum cyminum*) is another invaluable herb for digestive health. Its warming nature supports Agni, enhancing the digestive process and reducing indigestion. Cumin also aids in the absorption of nutrients and possesses antioxidant properties, protecting the digestive tract from damage. It's widely used in various cuisines and can be incorporated easily into daily meals. Ground cumin can be added to vegetable dishes, stews, or used as a spice in meat preparations. However, individuals with Pitta dosha should use cumin sparingly, given its warming nature.

Aloe vera (*Aloe barbadensis miller*) is a well-known herb with soothing and cooling properties, which makes it useful in treating inflammatory bowel conditions and other issues involving digestive discomfort such as ulcers or gastritis. Its gel is directly applied to affected areas, either orally or topically, in some cases. It has cooling effects, which aids in reducing inflammation and promoting healing within the digestive tract. It is best to consult a practitioner before using aloe vera for this purpose because of its potential laxative effect.

Beyond these specific herbs, Ayurveda offers a vast array of other herbal remedies tailored to address various digestive imbalances. For instance, coriander (*Coriandrum sativum*) is known for its ability to soothe the digestive tract and alleviate indigestion. Cardamom (*Elettaria cardamomum*) offers a delightful flavor and contributes to improving appetite and digestion. These herbs, among many others, highlight Ayurveda's holistic approach to health, addressing not only the symptoms of digestive issues but also their underlying causes.

However, it is critical to emphasize that self-treating with herbs can be risky. It is crucial to consult a qualified

Ayurvedic practitioner before using any herbal remedies, especially if you are pregnant, breastfeeding, or have pre-existing health conditions. A practitioner can assess your individual dosha, identify the root cause of your digestive problems, and recommend the most appropriate herbs and dosages for your unique needs.

Furthermore, the proper preparation and administration of herbal remedies are essential for their efficacy and safety. Some herbs require specific cooking methods to maximize their therapeutic benefits, while others are best consumed in specific forms, such as tinctures, capsules, or teas. A qualified practitioner can guide you on the best methods of preparing and using herbal remedies to ensure optimal results.

The integration of herbal remedies into a comprehensive Ayurvedic approach to digestive health maximizes their effectiveness. They are not a replacement for a healthy diet, mindful eating practices, or stress management techniques but rather valuable tools to further enhance the restoration of digestive balance. Remember that consistent application of these tools, coupled with a holistic lifestyle, is essential for long-term improvements in digestive health. The journey towards optimal digestive health is an ongoing process of self-awareness, mindful choices, and seeking professional guidance when needed.

Moreover, the understanding of the six tastes—sweet, sour, salty, pungent, bitter, and astringent—is also paramount in effectively using herbal remedies. The proper balance of these tastes within a meal plan and the consideration of an herb's specific taste are vital to its effectiveness and the overall balance of the doshas. A practitioner can help you understand how these tastes interact with your digestive system and how to use them to best support your unique constitution.

It's also important to remember that the effectiveness of herbal remedies can vary depending on factors such as the quality of the herbs, their processing, and the individual's response. Purchasing herbs from reputable sources, ensuring proper storage, and paying close attention to your body's response are crucial aspects of utilizing herbal remedies effectively and safely. Keeping a journal of your experience with these remedies, including their effects and any potential side effects, can be valuable in providing feedback to your practitioner and helping you fine-tune your personalized approach.

The use of herbal remedies should not overshadow the importance of addressing the root causes of digestive issues. Factors such as stress, poor sleep, irregular eating habits, and emotional imbalances can significantly impact digestive health. Integrating Ayurvedic practices such as yoga, meditation, and pranayama alongside herbal remedies can synergistically enhance digestive well-being and address these underlying factors. These practices help calm the nervous system, reduce stress, and foster a balanced internal environment that supports optimal digestion.

Finally, it is important to emphasize that Ayurvedic herbal remedies are not a quick fix. They often require consistent usage over time to achieve noticeable improvements in digestive health. Patience, self-awareness, and a holistic approach are crucial elements in the journey towards achieving optimal digestive health. Working closely with a qualified Ayurvedic practitioner ensures personalized guidance, safety, and effective outcomes, ultimately empowering you to achieve sustained digestive wellness and overall well-being. Through a combination of dietary changes, lifestyle adjustments, and the strategic use of herbal remedies, you can embark on a transformative journey toward a healthier, more vibrant you.

Lifestyle Practices to Support Healthy Digestion

Beyond the realm of diet and herbal remedies, the cornerstone of healthy digestion in Ayurveda lies in cultivating a lifestyle that nurtures and supports the digestive fire, or *Agni*. This involves a harmonious blend of mindful practices that extend beyond the kitchen and into every facet of daily life. Stress, for instance, is a significant Agni disruptor. The constant activation of the sympathetic nervous system, the body's "fight-or-flight" response, diverts energy away from digestion, leaving the body struggling to process food efficiently. Chronic stress leads to the accumulation of *Ama*, the toxic byproduct of improper digestion, which further weakens Agni and sets the stage for a cascade of health problems.

Effective stress management is therefore paramount. Ayurveda offers a variety of techniques to combat stress and promote relaxation, fostering a balanced state conducive to optimal digestion. Practicing yoga and pranayama (breathing exercises) are highly recommended. Specific asanas (yoga postures) like *Paschimottanasana* (seated forward bend) and *Bhujangasana* (cobra pose) gently massage the abdominal organs, stimulating peristalsis and improving digestion. Pranayama techniques such as *Dirga Pranayama* (three-part breath) and *Ujjayi Pranayama* (victorious breath) calm the nervous system, promoting relaxation and reducing stress hormones. These practices not only directly benefit digestion but also create a more balanced internal environment where Agni can thrive.

Meditation, another cornerstone of Ayurvedic stress management, quiets the mind and fosters a state of inner peace. Regular meditation practice, even for 10-15 minutes daily, can significantly reduce stress levels, improving sleep quality and enhancing the body's ability to digest food effectively. Mindfulness practices, such as paying attention to the sensations of eating, savoring each bite, and chewing food thoroughly, further enhance the digestive process by promoting better enzyme secretion and nutrient absorption. By cultivating a mindful awareness of our bodies and our responses to stress, we pave the way for improved digestive function.

Regular physical activity is another indispensable component of a digestive-supportive lifestyle. While vigorous exercise might be counterproductive immediately after a large meal, moderate activity throughout the day enhances circulation and aids in the movement of food through the digestive tract. Gentle walks, light stretching, and yoga are ideal choices; they promote lymphatic drainage, helping to eliminate toxins and improve overall digestive efficiency. The type and intensity of exercise should be tailored to individual dosha constitution. Vata individuals, characterized by their airy and mobile nature, might benefit from gentler forms of movement such as walking or yoga, avoiding intense workouts that could exacerbate their tendency towards dryness and imbalance. Pitta individuals, known for their fiery and energetic disposition, might need to adjust their workout intensity to prevent overheating and digestive upset. Kapha individuals, characterized by their stable and grounded nature, can benefit from more vigorous exercises to stimulate their metabolism and prevent sluggish digestion.

Sleep, often overlooked, is a critical factor in supporting healthy digestion. During sleep, the body undertakes vital restorative processes, including digestion and elimination. Insufficient or poor-quality sleep disrupts these processes, leading to digestive imbalances. Ayurveda emphasizes the importance of a regular sleep schedule, aiming for 7-8 hours of uninterrupted sleep each night. Establishing a consistent bedtime routine, creating a relaxing bedtime environment, and avoiding caffeine and alcohol before bed can significantly improve sleep quality and indirectly support healthy digestion. The darkness of night plays a significant role in the body's production of melatonin, a hormone that regulates sleep-wake cycles. Exposure to artificial light in the evenings can disrupt this natural process, affecting sleep and ultimately digestion.

Another crucial aspect of lifestyle for optimal digestion is maintaining regularity in bowel movements. Constipation is a common digestive issue that contributes to the accumulation of Ama and weakens Agni. Ayurveda recommends several strategies to promote healthy elimination. Adequate hydration is crucial; drinking ample amounts of water throughout the day helps to soften the stool and facilitates its passage through the intestines. Including fiber-rich foods in the diet, such as fruits, vegetables, and whole grains, adds bulk to the stool, stimulating peristalsis and promoting regularity. Regular physical activity, as discussed earlier, also aids in bowel movements by stimulating the muscles of the digestive tract. Abdominal massage, either self-administered or by a therapist, can gently stimulate peristalsis and relieve constipation.

Beyond these foundational practices, Ayurveda emphasizes the importance of mindful living and maintaining a positive mental outlook. Emotions like anger, frustration, and worry can significantly disrupt digestion, affecting Agni and contributing to the formation of Ama. Practices that promote emotional well-being, such as meditation, spending time in nature, engaging in hobbies, and connecting with loved ones, are crucial for maintaining a balanced state and supporting healthy digestion. Cultivating gratitude and practicing forgiveness can also promote emotional harmony and improve overall digestive health. These practices encourage a sense of inner peace and tranquility, creating a favorable environment for optimal digestive function.

The timing of meals also plays a significant role in digestive health. Ayurveda recommends eating at regular intervals, avoiding both excessive skipping of meals and excessive overeating. It's crucial to consume meals when Agni is strong, typically during the midday and early evening hours. Avoid eating late at night, as digestion slows down during sleep, hindering the body's ability to process food properly. Eating in a calm and relaxed environment, free from distractions, allows for proper digestion and nutrient absorption. Mindful eating, focusing on the taste, texture, and aroma of food, promotes better enzyme secretion and enhances satiety, preventing overeating. By paying attention to the timing and atmosphere of our meals, we can create an environment conducive to optimal digestion.

Incorporating these lifestyle practices into daily life requires dedication and commitment, but the rewards are significant. By addressing the underlying factors that influence digestion, we not only improve our digestive health but also enhance our overall well-being. These practices are not isolated interventions; they are interconnected aspects of a holistic approach to health and wellness, reflecting the interconnectedness that Ayurveda recognizes between the mind, body, and spirit. Consistent application of these principles cultivates a resilient digestive system, strengthening Agni, reducing Ama, and paving the way for a healthier, more vibrant life. The journey towards optimal digestive health is a continuous process of learning, adapting, and refining our lifestyle choices to better align with the principles of Ayurveda and our individual constitution. Remember that patience and self-compassion are essential components of this journey. It's not about perfection, but about consistent progress toward a healthier and more balanced you. By embracing these practices, you are investing not only in your digestive health but in your overall well-being, creating a foundation for a life filled with vitality and joy. The holistic approach of Ayurveda offers a path towards sustainable health, empowering individuals to take charge of their well-being and experience the profound benefits of a balanced life.

A Comprehensive Guide

Embarking on your 30-day Ayurvedic wellness journey is a commitment to nurturing your mind, body, and spirit. This plan, divided into four weeks, provides a structured approach to integrating Ayurvedic principles into your daily life. Remember, consistency is key. Don't strive for perfection; focus on progress and gentle self-compassion. Each week builds upon the previous one, gradually deepening your understanding and practice. Adapt this plan to suit your individual needs and dosha, and always listen to your body's wisdom.

Week 1: Establishing a Foundation

This first week focuses on laying a solid foundation for your Ayurvedic journey. We'll concentrate on establishing consistent daily routines (Dinacharya), introducing balanced meals, and incorporating gentle movement. The emphasis here is on building healthy habits rather than drastic changes.

Dietary Focus:
Begin by focusing on easily digestible foods, minimizing processed foods, refined sugars, and excessive caffeine. Prioritize whole grains like brown rice and quinoa, plenty of fresh fruits and vegetables, and lean proteins. If you are Vata, focus on warming foods like soups and stews. If you are Pitta, opt for cooling foods like cucumber and coconut water. If you are Kapha, incorporate lighter, warming spices like ginger and turmeric. Pay attention to the six tastes – sweet, sour, salty, pungent, bitter, and astringent – ensuring a balance in your meals. Avoid overeating, and practice mindful eating, savoring each bite.

Exercise:
Begin with gentle exercise like walking for 20-30 minutes daily. If you enjoy yoga, practice gentle stretches and sun salutations. Listen to your body and avoid strenuous activity, especially during the early days. The goal is to gently awaken your body and promote circulation.

Dinacharya:
Establish a consistent morning and evening routine. Start your day with a glass of warm water with lemon, followed by tongue scraping and oil pulling. In the evening, wind down with a warm bath or shower, and practice a calming meditation or breathing exercise (pranayama). Aim for 7-8 hours of quality sleep. Adjust your routine based on your dosha. A Vata individual might benefit from a more structured routine, while a Kapha individual might need to incorporate more invigorating activities into their morning routine.

Self-Care:
Incorporate self-massage (Abhyanga) using warm sesame oil (for Vata), coconut oil (for Pitta), or almond oil (Kapha) at least twice a week. This simple act of self-love will help to nourish your skin and calm your nervous system. Spend some time each day in nature, whether it's a short walk in a park or simply sitting under a tree.

Week 2: Deepening the Practice

In the second week, we'll delve deeper into your Ayurvedic practice. We'll refine your dietary choices, introduce more challenging exercises, and incorporate specific Ayurvedic techniques for stress management.

Dietary Focus:
Continue with the balanced diet from week one, but start incorporating more variety. Experiment with new dosha-specific recipes, and pay closer attention to how different foods affect your energy levels and digestion.

Introduce more spices to enhance the taste and therapeutic benefits of your meals. For instance, cumin and coriander are beneficial for digestion, while ginger helps to reduce inflammation.

Exercise:
Gradually increase the intensity and duration of your exercise. If you are practicing yoga, you can begin to incorporate more challenging asanas. Consider adding other forms of light to moderate exercise, like swimming or cycling. Always listen to your body, and never push yourself beyond your limits.

Dinacharya:
Refine your daily routine based on your experiences from the first week. Pay close attention to the timing of your meals and your sleep schedule. Experiment with different pranayama techniques to see what works best for you.

Stress Management:
Introduce a daily mindfulness or meditation practice. Even 10-15 minutes of quiet contemplation can have a significant impact on your stress levels. Practice deep breathing exercises to help regulate your nervous system. Explore aromatherapy using calming essential oils like lavender or chamomile.

Week 3: Integrating Advanced Practices

During the third week, we will explore more advanced Ayurvedic practices to further enhance your well-being. This might include incorporating specific herbal remedies or exploring gentle detoxification techniques.

Dietary Focus:
Continue to refine your diet, focusing on seasonal foods and reducing any foods that trigger imbalances. Experiment with different food combinations to optimize digestion. Consider incorporating Ayurvedic herbal

teas to support your digestive health. For example, ginger tea can soothe an upset stomach, while fennel tea can help relieve bloating.

Exercise:
Maintain a regular exercise routine, but incorporate variety to prevent boredom. Try a new type of yoga, or incorporate other forms of exercise like dancing or Tai Chi. Remember to listen to your body and rest when needed.

Dinacharya:
Further refine your daily routine, paying close attention to the timing of your meals, exercise, and sleep. Ensure that your routine aligns with your natural circadian rhythm.

Advanced Practices:
Introduce gentle detoxification techniques such as oil pulling or a short, simple cleanse, always under the guidance of a qualified health professional. Explore the use of specific Ayurvedic herbs under the supervision of a knowledgeable practitioner. Remember that herbal remedies should be used cautiously and only after consultation with a professional.

Week 4: Sustaining Your Wellness

The final week is about consolidating your progress and creating a sustainable Ayurvedic lifestyle. We'll focus on maintaining your healthy habits and transitioning smoothly into a long-term commitment to your well-being.

Dietary Focus:
By this point, you should have a good understanding of which foods nourish you and which ones cause imbalances. Continue to prioritize whole, unprocessed foods, and minimize those that trigger negative reactions. Maintain a balanced intake of all six tastes.

Exercise:
Continue your regular exercise routine, focusing on sustainability. Find activities you enjoy and that fit easily into your lifestyle. Don't feel pressured to maintain a rigorous schedule; consistency is more important than intensity.

Dinacharya:
Your daily routine should now be well-established. Continue to prioritize sleep, mindful eating, and stress-reducing activities. Adjust your routine as needed to accommodate changes in your life and your energy levels.

Long-term Plan:
This week is about reflecting on your progress and creating a plan for maintaining your Ayurvedic lifestyle long-term. Identify any challenges you faced and develop strategies for overcoming them. Consider ways to incorporate Ayurvedic principles into all aspects of your life.

Remember, Ayurveda is a journey, not a destination. This 30-day plan is just the beginning. Be patient with yourself, celebrate your progress, and continue to learn and grow. With consistent effort and mindful practice, you will cultivate a deeper understanding of your body and its needs, leading to a healthier, happier, and more balanced life. Remember to consult with a qualified Ayurvedic practitioner or registered dietitian for personalized guidance, especially if you have any underlying health conditions. They can help you tailor the plan to your specific needs and ensure your safety.

Delicious and Nutritious Recipes

Now that we've laid the groundwork for your 30-day Ayurvedic journey, let's delve into the delicious and nourishing meals that will fuel your transformation. Remember, the key to Ayurvedic eating lies in balancing the six tastes: sweet, sour, salty, bitter, pungent, and astringent. Each taste has specific properties and affects the doshas differently. A balanced diet incorporates all six tastes in moderation, ensuring equilibrium within your system.

Week 1: Establishing Balance

This week focuses on establishing a foundation of healthy eating habits. We'll prioritize easily digestible foods that gently cleanse and nourish the body. The emphasis is on warming, grounding foods for all doshas, providing a solid base for the weeks to come.

Day 1-7 Sample Meal Plan (adaptable to all doshas):
Breakfast:
Warm oatmeal with a sprinkle of cinnamon and a handful of berries. (Adaptable: Vata can add ghee; Pitta can add a squeeze of lemon; Kapha can add a touch of nutmeg.)
Lunch:
Lentil soup (dal) with brown rice and a side of
steamed vegetables like spinach or carrots. (Adaptable: Vata can add warming spices like ginger and cumin; Pitta can opt for a lighter broth; Kapha can add a pinch of black pepper.)
Dinner:
Roasted root vegetables (sweet potatoes, carrots, parsnips) with a side of quinoa and a small amount of grilled chicken or fish. (Adaptable: Vata can add a drizzle of sesame oil; Pitta can add cilantro; Kapha can add a squeeze of lime.)
Snacks:
A small handful of almonds or walnuts, a piece of fruit

(apple, pear, banana), or a small bowl of vegetable sticks with hummus.

Week 2: Deepening the Practice

As you settle into your routine, we'll introduce more variety and complexity to your meals. This week emphasizes incorporating a wider range of spices and herbs to enhance digestion and support your individual dosha.

Day 8-14 Sample Meal Plan (dosha-specific examples):

Vata:
Breakfast:
Warm milk with cardamom and a touch of honey. Kitcheri (a mung bean and rice porridge) with ghee.
Lunch:
Steamed vegetables with brown rice and a lentil stew seasoned with ginger and cumin.
Dinner:
Sweet potato and chickpea curry with basmati rice. **Snacks:** Dates, warm almond milk, sunflower seeds.

Pitta:
Breakfast:
Porridge made with barley or quinoa, topped with coconut flakes and berries.
Lunch:
Cucumber and mint raita (yogurt dip) with brown rice and grilled vegetables.
Dinner:
Steamed fish with asparagus and zucchini.
Snacks:
Coconut water, watermelon, a small amount of avocado.

Kapha:
Breakfast:
Spiced apple and cinnamon smoothie (with almond milk).
Lunch:
Lentil salad with a light vinaigrette and mixed greens.

Dinner:
Roasted vegetables with quinoa and a small amount of lean protein (chicken or tofu).
Snacks:
Green tea, a small amount of berries, a handful of lightly roasted chickpeas.

Week 3: Exploring Seasonal Flavors

This week introduces the concept of seasonal eating, an essential aspect of Ayurvedic wellness. We'll focus on foods that are in season and best suited to your dosha and the current climate. (Note: This section would need to be adjusted based on the time of year the book is being read.) For example, in the summer, lighter, cooling foods are emphasized, while in the winter, warm, grounding foods are preferred.

Day 15-21 Sample Meal Plan (example for late Summer):

Vata:
Emphasize warm, cooked meals with grounding spices. Consider adding more warming soups and stews.
Pitta:
Focus on cooling foods like cucumber, watermelon, and mint. Incorporate light, easily digestible meals.
Kapha:
Prioritize lighter meals, increase the consumption of bitter and pungent spices, and include more leafy greens.

Week 4: Integrating Ayurvedic Principles

The final week integrates all the principles learned throughout the month. This week encourages you to experiment with different recipes and combinations, tailoring your meals to your individual needs and preferences while remaining mindful of your dosha.

Day 22-28 Sample Meal Plan (Recipes and variations):

Recipe 1: Simple Kitchari (adaptable to all doshas):
1 cup basmati rice, 1 cup yellow mung dal (split mung beans), 6 cups water, 1 tsp ghee, 1 tsp cumin seeds, 1/2 tsp turmeric powder, 1/4 tsp ginger powder, salt to taste. Combine all ingredients except ghee and salt in a pot, bring to a boil, and

simmer until the rice and dal are cooked and mushy. Add ghee and salt to taste.

Recipe 2: Spiced Carrot and Chickpea Curry (Vata and Kapha balancing):

1 tbsp olive oil, 1 onion (chopped), 2 carrots (diced), 1 can chickpeas (drained and rinsed), 1 tsp cumin seeds, 1/2 tsp turmeric powder, 1/4 tsp coriander powder, 1/4 tsp garam masala, salt and pepper to taste. Sautéonion in oil, add spices and cook for a minute. Add carrots and chickpeas, cook until carrots are tender. Season to taste. Serve with brown rice or quinoa.

Recipe 3: Cooling Cucumber Raita (Pitta balancing):

1 cup plain yogurt, 1 cucumber (grated), 1/4 cup chopped mint, 1/4 tsp cumin powder, salt to taste. Combine all ingredients and mix well.

Recipes for each Dosha (expanded examples):

To further illustrate the principles of dosha-specific cooking, let's provide more detailed examples. These are just starting points; feel free to adapt them to your preferences and the ingredients available to you. Remember to always prioritize fresh, organic ingredients whenever possible.

Vata-Pacifying Recipes:

Vata-Pacifying Soup:

This hearty soup combines warming spices and root vegetables to ground and stabilize Vata energy. Ingredients: 1 tbsp ghee, 1 onion (chopped), 2 carrots (diced), 2 parsnips (diced), 4 cups vegetable broth, 1 tsp ginger powder, 1/2 tsp cumin powder, 1/4 tsp coriander powder, salt and pepper to taste. Sauté onion in ghee, add spices and cook for a minute. Add carrots, parsnips, and broth. Simmer until vegetables are tender. Season to taste.

Warm Millet Porridge:

This easily digestible breakfast provides sustained energy and nourishment. Ingredients: 1/2 cup millet, 2 cups water, 1/4 cup milk (almond or cow's milk), 1 tsp ghee, a pinch of cardamom. Cook millet in water until tender. Stir in milk and ghee. Add cardamom.

Pitta-Balancing Recipes:

Cooling Cucumber Salad:

This refreshing salad helps to cool down and pacify Pitta's fiery nature. Ingredients: 1 cucumber (sliced), 1/2 cup chopped cilantro, 1/4 cup lime juice, 1/4 tsp cumin powder, salt to taste. Combine all ingredients and mix well.

Light Lentil Soup:

This light and easily digestible soup provides essential nutrients without overwhelming the digestive system. Ingredients: 1 cup red lentils, 4 cups water, 1/2 cup chopped spinach, 1/4 cup chopped cilantro, salt and pepper to taste. Cook lentils in water until soft. Stir in spinach and cilantro. Season to taste.

Kapha-Reducing Recipes:

Spiced Green Beans:

This dish incorporates pungent spices to stimulate digestion and reduce Kapha accumulation.
Ingredients: 1 lb green beans (trimmed), 1 tbsp olive oil, 1/2 tsp mustard seeds, 1/4 tsp cumin seeds, 1/4 tsp turmeric powder, a pinch of red pepper flakes, salt and pepper to taste. Sauté mustard and cumin seeds in oil. Add green beans, spices, and salt. Cook until tender-crisp. Season to taste.

Light Vegetable Stir-fry:

This quick and easy stir-fry provides a variety of nutrients without being too heavy.

Ingredients: 1 tbsp sesame oil, assortment of vegetables (broccoli, carrots, peppers, zucchini), 1/4 tsp ginger powder, 1/4 tsp garlic powder, soy sauce (tamari for gluten-free), salt and pepper to taste. Stir-fry vegetables in oil until tender-crisp. Add spices and soy sauce. Season to taste.

Week 5: Maintaining Your Ayurvedic Balance

This is not a week of new recipes, but rather a continuation of the principles and practices already established. It's a crucial time to reflect on your journey and adjust your plan accordingly. You may discover certain foods work better for you than others, or your preferences may shift as the weeks progress. This flexibility is a key component of Ayurvedic living. Continue to prioritize the six tastes and ensure a balance of them within your diet. Listen to your body's cues, and don't hesitate to tweak your recipes and meal timings to suit your individual needs. This adaptable approach is paramount to establishing a sustainable, long-term practice. Remember that this 30-day plan is merely a springboard to a holistic lifestyle. The real work begins now. Continue to experiment with new recipes and variations, always focusing on seasonal ingredients and creating nourishing meals that support your individual dosha and overall well-being.

This 30-day plan offers a structured approach, but remember, flexibility is key. Listen to your body's intuitive wisdom; Ayurveda is a deeply personal practice, and there is no one-size-fits-all approach. This individualized journey of self-discovery is the core of Ayurveda's enduring appeal.

Cultivating Balance Through Routine

The foundation of a successful 30-day Ayurvedic wellness plan rests not just on mindful eating, but also on the consistent practice of daily routines, known as Dinacharya. Think of Dinacharya as the scaffolding that supports your Ayurvedic lifestyle, providing a structure for maintaining balance and preventing imbalances from arising in the first place. This daily regimen is not a rigid set of rules, but rather a personalized framework tailored to your individual dosha and lifestyle, designed to harmonize with your body's natural rhythms. It's about cultivating a sense of mindful awareness and aligning your actions with the natural world.

The beauty of Dinacharya lies in its simplicity and adaptability. The practices are easily incorporated into even the busiest of schedules, and the benefits are profound. By establishing a consistent daily routine, you create a sense of order and predictability, reducing stress and promoting a feeling of calm and centeredness. This, in turn, allows your body to function optimally, strengthening your digestive fire (Agni), boosting immunity, and enhancing overall well-being. Consistent practice is key; even small, consistent efforts will yield significant results over time.

Let's start with the cornerstone of Dinacharya: waking up with the sun. Aim to rise before sunrise, ideally between 6:00 am and 6:30 am. This aligns with the natural rhythms of the body and allows you to begin your day with a sense of calm and intention. The quality of your morning sets the tone for the rest of your day. Avoid hitting the snooze button; this can disrupt your natural sleep cycle and leave you feeling groggy and disoriented. Instead, gently rouse yourself, perhaps with a soft melody or the gentle sounds of nature.

Upon waking, gently cleanse your tongue with a tongue scraper. This removes toxins that accumulate overnight, promoting better oral hygiene and improving your sense of taste. Follow this with warm water, perhaps with a squeeze of fresh lemon. This helps stimulate digestion and cleanses the digestive tract. Avoid cold water, especially if you have a Vata dosha, as it can aggravate the Vata element and lead to digestive discomfort.

Next, attend to your elimination needs. Regular bowel movements are crucial for removing waste products and maintaining a healthy digestive system. If you experience constipation, consider incorporating fiber-rich foods into your diet, increasing water intake, and gentle exercise. Ayurveda emphasizes the importance of regularity in elimination – a healthy bowel movement in the morning is a sign of a balanced system.

After eliminating, engage in a gentle self-massage, known as Abhyanga. This practice uses warm, preferably sesame, coconut, or almond oil to massage your body. The massage stimulates circulation, nourishes the skin, and relaxes the nervous system. Each dosha benefits from Abhyanga, but the oil choice should be adjusted according to your individual constitution. Vata doshas might benefit from more warming oils, while Pitta doshas might prefer cooling oils.

Following Abhyanga, a warm shower or bath is recommended. Avoid excessively hot water, as this can deplete your energy. Instead, opt for a lukewarm shower, and consider adding a few drops of essential oils, such as lavender or chamomile, for relaxation and aromatherapy benefits. The shower or bath should be a sensory experience, allowing you to transition fully into your day.

Now, it's time for your daily meditation or prayer. Even 10-15 minutes of mindful meditation or a moment of prayer can have a profoundly positive impact on your mental and emotional well-being. This practice can help calm the mind, reduce stress, and increase self-awareness. Choose a technique that resonates with you, whether it's guided meditation, mindfulness practices, or simply focusing on your breath.

Next, turn your attention to your morning meal. As discussed in the previous chapter, this should be a nourishing and balanced meal that supports your dosha. Remember the six tastes: sweet, sour, salty, bitter, pungent, and astringent. Aim for a combination of these tastes to promote optimal digestion and energy levels. Avoid heavy, greasy, or overly spicy foods in the morning. A lighter meal allows for optimal digestion and prevents sluggishness throughout the day.

Throughout the day, maintain mindful awareness of your posture, whether sitting or standing. Good posture improves circulation, supports organ function, and reduces stress on the body. Integrate short breaks for mindful movement into your workday. A brief walk, stretching, or a few sun salutations can revitalize your body and mind, combating the effects of prolonged sitting.

Your midday meal should be your most substantial meal of the day, allowing ample time for digestion before you wind down for the evening. Again, choose a balanced meal incorporating the six tastes according to your dosha's requirements.

As the evening approaches, begin to slow down your pace. Prepare for a peaceful and restful night. In the late afternoon or early evening, engage in some form of light exercise, such as a gentle walk or yoga. Avoid strenuous activity close to bedtime, as it can interfere with sleep.

About an hour before bedtime, take a warm bath or shower to relax your muscles and prepare your body for sleep. Consider adding Epsom salts or essential oils to enhance the relaxing effects.

Before sleep, engage in a relaxing activity such as reading, listening to calming music, or practicing gentle stretching. Avoid screen time close to bedtime, as the blue light emitted from electronic devices can interfere with melatonin production, making it harder to fall asleep. Ensure your bedroom is dark, quiet, and cool to promote optimal sleep quality.

The practice of Dinacharya extends beyond specific actions; it's about cultivating a mindset of balance and self-awareness. It is a holistic approach to daily living, not simply a checklist of tasks. By aligning your actions with the natural rhythms of your body and the environment, you create a foundation for optimal health and well-being.

Stress management is an integral part of Dinacharya. In today's fast-paced world, stress is pervasive. Chronic stress disrupts the delicate balance of the doshas, leading to various health problems. Ayurveda offers a range of techniques for managing stress effectively. These techniques can be seamlessly integrated into your daily routine to enhance your resilience and promote a sense of inner peace.

Deep breathing exercises are a simple yet powerful way to reduce stress. Practicing deep, diaphragmatic breathing for even a few minutes can calm the nervous system and lower cortisol levels. Try the Ujjayi breath, or "ocean breath", where you gently constrict the back of your throat as you inhale and exhale, creating a soft, ocean-like sound. This deep breathing technique has calming and grounding effects.

Yoga and Pranayama are also excellent tools for stress management. Yoga postures (asanas) help to release tension from the muscles and improve flexibility, while Pranayama (breathing exercises) calm the mind and reduce stress hormones. Choose yoga styles that align with your dosha and energy level. Restorative yoga is particularly effective for stress reduction.

Meditation and mindfulness practices can help you become more aware of your thoughts and emotions, allowing you to manage stress more effectively. Regular meditation reduces stress, lowers blood pressure, and improves overall mental well-being. Spend time in nature to recharge.

Nature walks have a profound impact on mental and emotional well-being. Spend time in nature, connect with the earth, and allow yourself to feel grounded and calm. The natural world is inherently restorative, offering a break from the demands of daily life.

Prioritize sleep hygiene. Adequate sleep is vital for stress management. Aim for 7-8 hours of uninterrupted sleep each night. Maintain a consistent sleep schedule, even on weekends, to regulate your body's natural sleep-wake cycle.

Establish a healthy social support system. Connecting with loved ones and engaging in meaningful relationships is crucial for managing stress. A strong support network helps to buffer against stress and promotes emotional well-being.

Practice self-compassion. Be kind and gentle to yourself. Acknowledge your strengths and limitations, and treat yourself with the same compassion you would extend to a loved one. Self-compassion is a vital component of stress management.

By consistently incorporating these stress-management techniques into your daily routine, you will build resilience against stress and cultivate a sense of inner peace. Remember, the goal of Dinacharya is not perfection, but progress. Even small, consistent efforts will yield significant benefits over time. Embrace the journey of self-discovery and find what works best for you. Your 30-day Ayurvedic wellness plan is a personal voyage of self-care, and this daily practice is your compass.

Monitoring Your Wellbeing

The journey towards optimal well-being, as outlined in your 30-day Ayurvedic wellness plan, is a deeply personal one. It's not a race to the finish line, but a mindful exploration of your body's unique needs and responses. Tracking your progress is therefore not about achieving some arbitrary benchmark, but about cultivating a deeper understanding of yourself and how you interact with the world around you. This involves a blend of objective measurements and subjective observations, allowing you to gain valuable insights and make necessary adjustments along the way.

One of the most effective ways to monitor your progress is through consistent self-reflection. This involves dedicating a few minutes each day, perhaps before bed or upon waking, to assess how you feel. Ask yourself questions such as: How is my digestion? Am I experiencing any bloating, constipation, or diarrhea? Is my sleep restful and restorative, or is it disturbed and fragmented? How is my energy level throughout the day? Do I feel clear-headed and focused, or sluggish and mentally foggy? How's my mood? Am I experiencing irritability, anxiety, or depression? Note any changes in your skin, such as dryness, oiliness, or breakouts. These are all valuable indicators of your overall balance.

Consider keeping a journal to document your observations. This doesn't need to be a detailed scientific record, but rather a personal reflection on your daily experiences. You might use a simple format with prompts like the ones mentioned above, or create a more free-flowing diary entry. The key is consistency. The more consistently you record your observations, the clearer the patterns will emerge. This self-monitoring will reveal the efficacy of your Ayurvedic practices and help you understand your body's subtle cues. For example, if you notice a consistent increase in energy levels after incorporating a specific yoga sequence or dietary change, you'll know to continue or even expand upon that practice. Conversely, if you observe negative changes—such as increased anxiety after consuming certain foods—you can make informed adjustments to your plan.

Beyond subjective observation, consider incorporating some objective measurements into your tracking process. Weighing yourself regularly can provide insights into your weight management journey, but remember that weight alone isn't the sole indicator of well-being. It's more beneficial to observe trends rather than fixate on daily fluctuations. If you're consistently losing weight or gaining weight (depending on your goal), this could provide a clue about the effectiveness of your dietary choices. However, more significantly, it is crucial to focus on measurements that reflect overall health and balance rather than simply weight. Your waist circumference, for example, provides an indicator of visceral fat, which is linked to increased health risks. Regular blood pressure and blood sugar readings, when appropriate and if recommended by your healthcare provider, can offer further insights into your metabolic health. Again, consistency is key. Tracking these metrics over time allows you to see patterns and make necessary modifications to your plan.

The use of technology can also significantly aid in tracking your progress. Numerous apps are available to monitor your diet, exercise, sleep patterns, and mood. Many of these apps also offer features to track water intake, which is crucial for optimal health and digestion within the framework of Ayurvedic practices. Choose an app that suits your needs and preferences, and remember that the technology is a tool to assist you, not dictate your journey. Avoid becoming overly obsessed with the numbers; the focus should always remain on achieving holistic balance.

Incorporating mindfulness meditation into your daily routine can enhance your self-awareness and sensitivity to subtle shifts in your energy and well-being. Regular meditation allows you to observe your thoughts and emotions without judgment, which is crucial for identifying patterns and stressors that might be impacting your progress. This can aid in pinpointing potential imbalances before they become significant problems. For example, you might notice increased restlessness and anxiety during a period of increased stress at work. This awareness, gained through meditation, allows you to proactively implement stress-reduction techniques such as deep breathing exercises or restorative yoga, thereby maintaining your overall balance.

Beyond specific metrics and technological tools, pay attention to your overall sense of well-being. Are you experiencing increased clarity, focus, and contentment? Are your relationships improving? Do you feel more connected to yourself and the world around you? These are all signs that your Ayurvedic journey is bearing fruit. While physical improvements are important, the holistic approach of Ayurveda emphasizes the interconnectedness of mind, body, and spirit. Tracking your progress involves acknowledging and celebrating the positive changes in all aspects of your life.

Consider incorporating regular check-ins with a qualified Ayurvedic practitioner or healthcare professional. While this 30-day plan provides a structured framework, a personalized assessment by a professional can provide invaluable insights and guidance. They can help you fine-tune your plan, address any specific concerns, and provide support as you navigate your journey. Remember, this isn't a solitary endeavor. Seeking support from a professional is a sign of self-care and commitment to your holistic well-being.

Remember, setbacks are inevitable. There will be days when you deviate from your plan, or when you feel like your progress is stalled. This is perfectly normal. The key is not to beat yourself up over minor slip-ups, but to gently adjust your course and continue moving forward. Review your journal entries, reflect on what might have caused the setback, and identify strategies to prevent it from happening again. Perhaps you need to adjust your meal plan, incorporate more restorative practices, or address underlying stress. Each setback is an opportunity for growth and learning.

Throughout this 30-day plan, cultivate patience and self-compassion. The journey toward optimal well-being is a continuous process, not a destination. Celebrate your achievements, big and small, and acknowledge the effort you're putting into improving your health. Your consistent effort, coupled with mindful observation and adjustments, will lay the foundation for a lifetime of vibrant health and well-being. By actively tracking your progress, you are not only monitoring your physical and mental state, but also nurturing a deeper connection to yourself and your innate capacity for healing and balance. This self-awareness is a gift that will extend far beyond the 30-day plan, empowering you to live a more fulfilling and harmonious life. The information and techniques provided within this book are meant to guide and empower you; however, always consult with your healthcare professional for personalized advice and treatment. Remember that self-care is not selfish; it's essential for cultivating a life filled with vitality, joy, and purpose.

Beyond the physical indicators, pay close attention to your subtle energy levels, your prana. Ayurveda teaches that prana, or life force, flows through our bodies, impacting our vitality and overall sense of well-being. Are you feeling more energized and alive? Do you notice a greater sense of clarity and focus? Or do you still feel drained and sluggish despite following the plan? These subtle shifts in energy levels can provide valuable insights into your progress and the effectiveness of the practices. Note any changes in your sleep patterns, as sleep is crucial for restoring prana. Are you sleeping more soundly and waking up feeling refreshed, or are you still experiencing disturbed or fragmented sleep? If sleep remains an issue, consider adjusting your evening routine, reducing screen time before bed, or incorporating calming practices like pranayama (yogic breathing) into your bedtime routine.

Consider using a simple rating scale to track your overall sense of well-being. On a scale of 1 to 10, with 1 being the lowest and 10 being the highest, rate your overall energy levels, mood, sleep quality, digestion, and clarity of mind each day. This provides a quick and easy way to visualize your progress over time. Notice the trends and patterns that emerge. Do you notice a correlation between certain foods and your energy levels? Does your mood improve on days when you practice yoga or meditation? This self-assessment provides valuable data for fine-tuning your plan.

Finally, remember that this 30-day plan is just the beginning. It's an introduction to the principles and practices of Ayurveda, a journey of self-discovery that continues long after the 30 days are over. By establishing mindful habits, building self-awareness, and actively tracking your progress, you are laying the foundation for a lifetime of vibrant health and well-being. The knowledge and skills you acquire throughout this journey will empower you to navigate your health with greater understanding and confidence, fostering a deeper connection to your body and a more harmonious relationship with yourself and the world around you.

Transitioning Beyond the Plan

The completion of your 30-day Ayurvedic wellness plan marks not an end, but a significant milestone on your journey towards lasting well-being. This plan has served as a foundational stepping stone, providing you with a taste of Ayurvedic principles and practices tailored to your unique doshic constitution. Now, the focus shifts from structured adherence to a program to integrating these practices seamlessly into your everyday life, building a sustainable, personalized Ayurvedic lifestyle. This transition requires a mindful and gradual approach, avoiding the pitfall of abruptly abandoning the beneficial routines you've established.

One of the most crucial aspects of transitioning successfully is cultivating self-awareness. The 30-day plan provided a framework for observing your body's responses to dietary changes, exercise routines, and stress management techniques. Continue this practice. Maintain a journal, noting your energy levels, digestive health, sleep patterns, and emotional well-being. Identify what worked exceptionally well, what needed adjustments, and what perhaps wasn't the right fit for you. This ongoing self-assessment is vital for customizing your Ayurvedic journey, making it uniquely yours and ensuring its long-term sustainability.

Dietary adjustments are often the most challenging aspect of adopting a new lifestyle. The 30-day plan likely introduced you to specific dosha-balancing foods and recipes. The key now is not to revert to old eating habits but to gradually incorporate these beneficial foods into your regular diet. Start by identifying one or two meals per day where you can maintain the principles learned during the program. Perhaps breakfast continues to be a focus on warm porridge or a lighter dosha-balancing option, while lunch incorporates more seasonal vegetables and mindful portion control. Experiment with new recipes based on what you've learned, but allow flexibility and don't feel pressured to be perfect. Remember, Ayurveda is not about restriction, but about mindful choices that nourish your body and mind.

Consider preparing a weekly meal plan that incorporates the principles you have learned. This doesn't require rigid adherence, but rather a thoughtful approach to incorporating the six tastes into your meals, ensuring balance and avoiding excessive indulgence in any one taste. Remember that the ratio of tastes in your meals can shift based on the season and your individual needs. During the warmer months, you may need to reduce the amount of warming spices and increase the presence of cooling elements. This thoughtful seasonal awareness can significantly improve the effectiveness of your dietary choices.

Exercise, a cornerstone of Ayurvedic well-being, needs to be seamlessly integrated into your daily routine. The 30-day plan may have included specific yoga asanas or other forms of exercise suitable for your dosha. Instead of viewing exercise as a chore, think about incorporating it in ways that feel natural and enjoyable. A morning walk, a brisk cycle in the afternoon, or a mindful yoga session before bed – these small changes can build a sustainable exercise practice. Experiment with different activities to find what resonates with your body and your busy schedule. Avoid aiming for high-intensity workouts every day; prioritize consistent, moderate exercise that supports your overall well-being, not an exhaustive fitness challenge.

The concept of Dinacharya, the daily routine, is paramount in Ayurvedic practice. Maintaining a consistent wake-up and sleep schedule, incorporating self-massage (Abhyanga), and oil pulling are significant elements in promoting balance and vitality. Incorporate these into your daily life gradually, observing which practices offer the greatest benefits. You may find that a 10-minute morning self-massage with warm sesame oil becomes a deeply enjoyable and rejuvenating practice, while oil pulling can become part of your daily oral hygiene routine. These practices, seemingly small, can contribute significantly to your overall sense of well-being.

Stress management, another key element of the 30-day plan, remains crucial. Prioritize stress-reduction techniques that work for you, whether it is meditation, spending time in nature, practicing Pranayama (breathing exercises), listening to calming music, or simply dedicating time for quiet reflection. These mindful practices aren't just tools for managing stress; they are integral to nourishing your emotional health, nurturing resilience, and preventing burnout.

The transition away from the structured 30-day plan doesn't mean abandoning the supportive community you might have found during that period. Seek out online forums, local Ayurvedic practitioners, or like-minded individuals who share your commitment to this holistic lifestyle. Sharing your experiences, seeking guidance, and drawing inspiration from others on a similar journey can provide valuable support and motivation, especially during times of challenge.

Remember that setbacks are inevitable. There will be days when you slip up, when your dietary choices deviate from your intentions, or when stress leads to a disruption of your routine. View these setbacks not as failures, but as learning opportunities. Analyze what might have triggered the deviation and gently correct your course, focusing on self-compassion and understanding rather than self-criticism.

This self-awareness is crucial to maintaining a long-term commitment to your well-being.

Over time, the principles and practices of Ayurveda should become integrated into your lifestyle, shaping your habits and choices. You may find yourself intuitively making healthier decisions, prioritizing self-care, and navigating daily challenges with increased resilience. Your connection with your body will deepen, and you will become more attuned to your unique needs and responses.

Beyond the 30-day plan, consider exploring further Ayurvedic practices. You might consider incorporating Rasayana therapies, focusing on rejuvenation and longevity, or delving deeper into Panchakarma, the Ayurvedic detoxification process under the guidance of a qualified practitioner. These advanced techniques, when appropriately applied, can further enhance your well-being and help maintain balance. However, remember to approach these practices with caution and only under the supervision of an experienced Ayurvedic practitioner.

Your Ayurvedic journey is a lifelong commitment, an ongoing exploration of self-discovery. It's a journey of mindful choices, mindful practices, and a deepening connection to your body, mind, and spirit. The 30-day plan was a starting point, a foundation upon which you can now build a vibrant, sustainable, and fulfilling Ayurvedic lifestyle that enhances your well-being and supports your overall health for years to come. Embrace the process, celebrate your successes, learn from your setbacks, and continue your journey towards optimal well-being with unwavering commitment and self-compassion. The knowledge you have gained is an empowering tool; use it wisely to create a life of balance, vitality, and inner peace. Remember to listen to your body, honor your individual needs, and adapt your

Ayurvedic practices to fit your life. It is your unique path, and the journey is as important as the destination.

Acknowledgments

This book would not have been possible without the support and guidance of one very special individual. I express my deepest gratitude to my wife, Cathy, who is the inspiration for me to research and seek out all of the holistic information that I have learned so far. I hope all that read this are inspired to not only look at this as a life long change but also to search out other areas and practices that can benefit them as well.
Many things that this world offers right now are not in align whit what our bodies need or want. May this start the path to a new future for everyone.

Appendix

This appendix contains supplemental information to enhance your understanding and application of the principles discussed in this book.

Appendix A: Detailed Herb Guide:

Amla (Indian Gooseberry)
: Rich in Vitamin C, supports immunity, improves digestion, and rejuvenates tissues.

Ashwagandha
: Adaptogen for stress relief, supports energy, stamina, and overall vitality.

Triphala
: Combination of three fruits (Amalaki, Bibhitaki, Haritaki); aids digestion, detoxification, and overall rejuvenation.

Brahmi (Bacopa)
: Enhances cognitive function, reduces anxiety, and improves mental clarity.

Tulsi (Holy Basil)
: Boosts immunity, relieves respiratory disorders, and promotes mental clarity.

Neem
: Detoxifies blood, supports skin health, and has antifungal and antibacterial properties.

Turmeric
: Anti-inflammatory, supports joint health, digestion, and overall immunity.

Guduchi (Tinospora Cordifolia)
: Boosts immunity, improves liver function, and acts as an anti-inflammatory agent.

Shatavari
: Supports female reproductive health, balances hormones, and nourishes tissues.

Haritaki
: Supports digestion, acts as a mild laxative, and aids in detoxification.

Bibhitaki
: Balances Kapha, aids in respiratory health, and detoxifies.

Guggul
: Promotes healthy cholesterol levels, supports joint health, and aids weight management.

Punarnava: Diuretic, supports kidney health, and helps reduce water retention.

Vidanga: Antimicrobial, antiparasitic, and supports digestion.

Amalaki: Antioxidant, rejuvenative for tissues, and aids digestion.

Manjistha: Blood purifier, supports skin health, and improves complexion.

Kutki: Detoxifies the liver, supports digestion, and acts as an anti-inflammatory.

Bhringaraj: Promotes hair growth, supports liver health, and acts as a rejuvenative.

Yashtimadhu (Licorice): Soothes respiratory and digestive systems, balances Pitta, and boosts immunity.

Arjuna: Cardiovascular tonic, supports heart health, and strengthens muscles.

Bilva (Bael): Balances Vata and Kapha, supports digestion, and relieves diarrhea.

Chandan (Sandalwood): Cooling agent, improves skin health, and calms the mind.

Dashmool: Combination of ten roots; reduces inflammation, strengthens the respiratory system, and balances Vata.

Gokshura (Tribulus Terrestris): Diuretic, supports kidney health, and enhances stamina.

Kalmegh: Detoxifies liver, improves digestion, and boosts immunity.

Musta: Balances Pitta, aids digestion, and supports menstrual health.

Pippali (Long Pepper)
: Improves digestion, enhances metabolism, and boosts respiratory health.

Kapikacchu (Mucuna Pruriens)
: Supports nervous system health and male reproductive function.

Shankhpushpi
: Enhances memory, reduces anxiety, and supports cognitive function.

Agaru (Aquilaria Agallocha)
: Calms the mind, promotes skin health, and balances Vata.

Jatamansi
: Relieves stress, promotes sleep, and supports nervous system health.

Daruharidra (Berberis Aristata)
: Improves liver function, supports skin health, and aids digestion.

Atibala
: Rejuvenative, supports muscular strength, and balances Vata.

Bhumi Amla
: Supports liver health and improves digestion.

Shankhapushpi
: See above.

Kantakari
: Supports respiratory health and reduces inflammation.

Vacha (Acorus Calamus)
: Improves cognitive function and aids digestion.

Ksheerabala
: Nourishing oil for nerves and joints.

Kutaja
: Treats diarrhea and supports gut health.

Katuki
: Detoxifies liver and supports digestion.

Krishna Jeeraka
: Supports digestion and aids respiratory health.

Lashuna (Garlic)
: Supports cardiovascular health and reduces cholesterol.

Lodhra
: Improves skin health and supports female reproductive health.

Mandukaparni
: Enhances cognitive function and supports skin health.

Shilajit
: Boosts energy, enhances stamina, and supports overall vitality.

Yarrow
: Anti-inflammatory, improves digestion, and supports skin health.
Abhrak Bhasma
: Strengthens respiratory system and improves vitality.
Mukta Bhasma
: Supports bone health and calms the mind.
Trivrit
: Acts as a purgative and supports detoxification. **Danti**
: Potent laxative and detoxifier.
Gokhru
: See above (Gokshura).
Patha
: Supports digestion and respiratory health.

Pushkarmool
: Relieves respiratory issues and reduces inflammation.
Rakta Chandan
: Cooling agent, improves skin health. **Vasa**
: Supports respiratory health and reduces inflammation.
Chandrashoor
: Rich in nutrients, supports digestion.
Deodar
: Anti-inflammatory, supports joint health.
Eranda (Castor)
: Laxative, supports joint health.
Ksheera Kakoli
: Rejuvenative and nourishing.
Madhuka
: Supports respiratory and digestive health.
Nagarmotha (Cyperus Rotundus)
: Supports digestion and metabolism.
Sarpagandha
: Reduces blood pressure and calms the mind. **Tagara**
: Supports sleep and calms the mind.
Aragvadha (Cassia Fistula)
: Laxative, supports skin health.
Dhanyak (Coriander)
: Improves digestion and detoxifies.
Jyotishmati
: Enhances memory and supports cognitive health.
Kakamachi
: Improves liver health and detoxification.
Katphala
: Reduces respiratory congestion.
Madhuyashti
: See Yashtimadhu (Licorice).
Nilotpala
: Cooling agent, supports respiratory and skin health.
Shringi
: Reduces cough and respiratory issues.
Sindoor
: Supports skin and blood health.
Vasa (Adhatoda Vasica)
: See above.

Duralabha
: Enhances vitality and balances doshas.
Ela (Cardamom)
: Improves digestion and relieves respiratory issues.
Karkatashrungi
: Supports respiratory health.
Kesar (Saffron)
: Enhances complexion, supports digestion, and boosts mood.
Masha (Black Gram)
: Nourishes tissues and improves strength.
Purnarnava
: See Punarnava.
Rakta Chandana
: See above (Rakta Chandan).

Tanduliyaka
: Nourishing and detoxifying.
Vatsanabha
: Used in detoxified form; balances doshas. **Bala**
: Strengthens muscles and supports immunity.
Chitrak
: Enhances digestion and supports metabolism.
Devdaru (Deodar)
: See above.
Dhanaka
: See Dhanyak.
Durva
: Nourishing and cooling.
Hingu (Asafoetida)
: Improves digestion and reduces bloating.
Indrayava
: Supports digestion and detoxification.
Jivaka
: Rejuvenative and nourishing.
Kachura
: Supports respiratory and digestive health.
Katphala
: See above.
Kokilaksha
: Enhances stamina and supports kidney health. **Krishna Tulsi**
: See Tulsi.
Kshirakakoli
: See Ksheera Kakoli.
Kumkuma
: See Kesar.
Lajjalu
: Supports wound healing and balances Pitta.
Latakaranja
: Supports liver health and detoxification. **Madhuka**
: See above.
Manjistha
: See above.

Appendix B: Sample Ayurvedic Meal Plans (Expanded):

Meal Plan for Vata Dosha

Goal:
Grounding and warming foods to calm Vata and promote balance.

Best Tastes:
Sweet, sour, salty.

Breakfast:
- Warm oatmeal cooked with almond milk, cinnamon, cardamom, and chopped dates.

- Herbal tea with ginger and licorice.

Mid-Morning Snack:
- A handful of soaked almonds or a ripe banana.

Lunch:
- Mung dal khichdi (rice and lentils cooked with ghee, cumin, and turmeric).
- Steamed sweet potato with a dash of Himalayan salt.
- Warm spiced carrot soup.

Afternoon Snack:
- Masala chai with almond milk and jaggery.

Dinner:
- Quinoa cooked with roasted vegetables (zucchini, squash, and carrots) and fresh ginger.
- Spinach sautéed in ghee with garlic and mustard seeds.
- A small bowl of kheer (rice pudding).

Meal Plan for Pitta Dosha

Goal:
Cooling and calming foods to reduce heat and maintain equilibrium.
Best Tastes:
Sweet, bitter, astringent.
Breakfast:

- Chia seed pudding with coconut milk, fresh blueberries, and a sprinkle of cinnamon.
- Mint or fennel tea.

Mid-Morning Snack:
- A pear or cucumber slices with a dash of lime.

Lunch:
- Quinoa salad with steamed asparagus, leafy greens, and avocado.
- Cooling cilantro-mint chutney.
- Coconut water.

Afternoon Snack:
- Fresh coconut chunks or pomegranate seeds.

Dinner:
- Moong dal with fresh coriander.
- Steamed broccoli and cauliflower with a drizzle of tahini.
- A small bowl of cucumber raita (yogurt with cucumber and mint).

Meal Plan for Kapha Dosha

Goal:
Light, warm, and spicy foods to stimulate metabolism and reduce heaviness.
Best Tastes:
Bitter, pungent, astringent.
Breakfast:

- Warm spiced apple stew with cloves, ginger, and cinnamon.
- A small cup of black tea with a pinch of cardamom.

Mid-Morning Snack:

- A few slices of roasted pumpkin seeds or sunflower seeds.

Lunch:

- Lentil soup with turmeric, cumin, and a hint of cayenne pepper.
- Steamed kale and Brussels sprouts.
- Pickled ginger slices.

Afternoon Snack:

- A small handful of spicy roasted chickpeas.

Dinner:

- Grilled zucchini and eggplant with a lemon-garlic dressing.
- Millet or barley pilaf with fresh parsley.
- A small cup of ginger-lemon tea.

General Meal Plan for Detoxification

Goal:
Light, easily digestible meals to cleanse the body and promote rejuvenation.
Breakfast:

- Warm lemon water followed by a bowl of stewed prunes or soaked figs.

Mid-Morning Snack:
- A small glass of fresh green juice (celery, cucumber, cilantro, and a pinch of ginger).

Lunch:
- Simple kitchari (mung dal and rice) cooked with cumin, turmeric, and coriander.
- A side of steamed zucchini or bottle gourd.

Afternoon Snack:
- Herbal detox tea with fennel, coriander, and cumin seeds.

Dinner:
- Clear vegetable soup with fresh ginger and garlic.
- A small serving of steamed spinach with a dash of lemon juice.

Seasonal Adjustments

- **Spring:**
Focus on light, detoxifying meals with bitter greens and spices like turmeric and fenugreek.
- **Summer:**
Include cooling foods like cucumber, coconut, and mint, with minimal spices.

- **Fall:**
Emphasize grounding and warm foods like root vegetables, soups, and stews.
- **Winter:**
Opt for warm, nourishing meals with ghee, spices, and hearty grains like quinoa and millet.

Glossary

Agni:
The digestive fire; the metabolic process responsible for transforming food into energy.

Ama:
Undigested food and toxins that accumulate in the body.

Ayurveda:
The traditional system of medicine originating in India, emphasizing the balance of mind, body, and spirit.

Dosha:
One of the three fundamental energies that govern the body and mind: Vata, Pitta, and Kapha.

Dinacharya:
The daily routine for optimal health and well-being.

Kapha:
One of the three doshas, characterized by earth and water elements; associated with stability, grounding, and structure.

Panchakarma:
The five main Ayurvedic detoxification procedures.

Pitta:
One of the three doshas, characterized by fire and water elements; associated with metabolism, transformation, and digestion.

Rasayana:
Ayurvedic rejuvenation therapies aimed at promoting longevity and vitality.

Vata:
One of the three doshas, characterized by air and ether elements; associated with movement, energy, and creativity.

References

Author Biography

Scott Johnsey is a wellness enthusiast that is always studying old and new methods of finding a way to make oneself healthy on all levels, physical, spiritual and emotional. After his wife's diagnosis with breast cancer in October of 2021, he has dedicated many hour of research to find all the ways that the body can heal itself. Ayurvedic medicine has been practiced for over 5000 years and now it is being backed by science in some studies. He hopes that learning to center your body and listen to it will help others to overcome issues that they are having. As with all diets and exercise, consult your doctor first before changing anything in your lifestyle and diet that could adversely affect your health.

www.ingramcontent.com/pod-product-compliance
Lightning Source LLC
Chambersburg PA
CBHW052142220526
45471CB00004B/1490